Testimonials for C(
Having in

MW00655321

"The doctor patient relationship hinges (......... .. build
relationships with inquiry based on empathy and curiosity, to understand people's
true feelings and make accurate diagnoses."

—John Toussaint, MD
Founder and Executive Chairman, Catalysis Inc.

"A quick and most resourceful read! Going beyond the medical agenda to ask what
patients want is fundamental, makes a difference and does not take a lot of time. Clinicians need to read this book. It will expand their thinking about how they relate to
patients resulting in improved communication and better outcomes."

—Ed Millermaier, MD, MBA, FACP Pivot Partnerships

"What every healthcare provider should know! As a practicing physician for more
than 20 years, I have worked continually to improve my communication skills. This
book is brilliant in its simplicity. Every provider will be able to implement these
practices immediately and impact the lives of their patients."

—Madhumita Murphy, MD, MSCI, MBA

"This book is a must read for all healthcare professionals. Best practices for *conversations worth having* are woven throughout this book utilizing evidence-based
strategies and engaging stories. The reader becomes a part of each story, learning
how to navigate conversations and reflecting on how past interactions might have
been reframed."

—Therese Jamison RN, DNP, ACNP-BC, Professor of Nursing
Lawrence Technological University

"If you hope to deliver patient-centred care, this book has to be on your must-read
list. Excellent examples, actionable steps, and clear direction on how to turn your
interactions in the healthcare setting into "conversations worth having". Reading
this book will make you a more effective and successful health practitioner."

—Dr. Troy McGowan, DClinDent (Perio)
Pacific Smiles Group, Australia

"Conversations Worth Having in Healthcare elevates conversations in healthcare
and beyond. While primarily focused on patient-provider interactions, this book
offers paradoxically simple yet transformational frameworks and practices that are
applicable in all areas of work and life. If you are ready to strengthen relationships,
results, and create more ease in your life, read this book!"

—Colette Herrick, Executive/Leadership
Healthcare Coach & Consultant, Insight Shift

Conversations Worth Having in Healthcare

*Boost Satisfaction & Quality
Using Appreciative Inquiry*

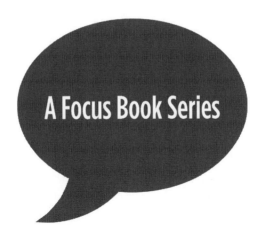

A Focus Book Series

Elizabeth Warner, MD and Fasiha Haq
with Cheri Torres and Jackie Stavros

CWH Publishers:
https://conversationsworthhaving.today
jackie@conversationsworthhaving.today
cheri@conversationsworthhaving.today

Cover Design and Graphics by Paul Stavros
Interior Formatting and Layout by Melissa Williams Design

ORDERING INFORMATION

Quantity sales. Special discounts are available on quantity purchases by corporations, associations, and others. For details, contact the "Special Sales Department" at the CWH Publishers.

Individual sales. CWH Publishers publications are available through Amazon and most bookstores.

Orders for college textbook/course adoption use. Please contact CWH Publishers.

This book is dedicated to those
who receive or deliver
healthcare.

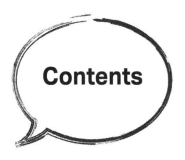

Contents

Acknowledgments

We would like to thank the following individuals for their support and contributions to this second book in our Focus Book Series for *Conversations Worth Having, Conversations Worth Having in Healthcare: Boost Satisfaction and Quality Using Appreciative Inquiry.*

First, we are grateful to our families for their support and encouragement.

Thanks to Colleen Watson for editorial expertise and advice, deep appreciation for Paul Stavros (our graphic genius!) who created our cover design, and Melissa Williams design who managed layout and design.

We are also grateful for those who read the manuscript offering feedback and testimonials for us. These include Philip Baer, Colette Herrick, Rakesh Jain, Therese Jamison, Troy McGowan, Ed Millermaier, Archana Mishra, Madhumita Murphy, Kim Thompson, John Toussaint, and Tim Vogus.

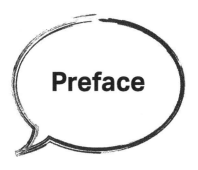

Preface

"We live in worlds our conversations create."

—*David Cooperrider*

Conversations are the heart of human interactions and effective healthcare. They can inspire us, improve outcomes, and foster wellbeing. They can also tear us apart, ruin our day, and increase distress. How often are you aware of your conversations? And how often are those *conversations worth having*?

I (Elizabeth Warner) have been an internal medicine physician and health system leader for over 20 years. My current work supports changing healthcare systems and energizing individuals who serve patients. While exploring Positive Organization Development, I studied Appreciative Inquiry (AI), and my worldview was forever changed. In focusing on what is good, positive, and possible in any interaction, my perspective has expanded, and possibilities have opened. In the book, *Conversations Worth Having: Using Appreciative Inquiry to Fuel Productive and Meaningful Engagement,* Jackie Stavros and Cheri Torres distill the power of AI into two communication practices. Applying these simple and elegant concepts has challenged me to communicate in new ways. This is true in healthcare conversations (e.g., with a patient and spouse having just received a terminal cancer diagnosis), in social interactions (e.g., at my high school reunion or with my sons at dinner), and in strategic discussions in the boardroom.

AI challenged my western medical training as a rational scientist. For all of my years of premed, medical school and residency training, advised to suppress emotional knowledge in favor of analytical thinking. I was taught to value linear, logical, reductionist, and procedural thinking. I was told that as physicians, we are special. I was indoctrinated into a medical care delivery system influenced by insurance companies and physician reimbursement structures built to reinforce the relative value of procedure over longitudinal care and human connection. These systems are insufficient to fully care for patients and healthcare professionals. We can do better, and I believe this book will help us do just that.

Having worked closely with physicians, patients, and a broad spectrum of healthcare providers across the globe for the past 30 years, I (Fasiha Haq) have experienced firsthand the complexities of navigating the healthcare ecosystem. Scientific research and technological advances have improved disease diagnosis, treatment, and care delivery. These same advances have also resulted in time and resource restrictions, administrative overload, and robotic processes in the name of efficiency. They impede empathetic communication and personal human connection, which is vital to enhancing the health and wellbeing of everyone involved.

Elevating both quality of care and access to care requires a multipronged approach that brings together diverse stakeholders in an open dialogue designed to broaden perspectives and collectively break through barriers that impede innovative healthcare solutions. Utilizing principles of neuroscience, behavioral science, positive psychology, and Appreciative Inquiry, I have developed and delivered multiple professional development initiatives designed to improve clinical performance. Healthcare professionals often express the need for resources that help bridge the disconnect amongst providers and patients and amongst interdisciplinary teams. They have been pleasantly surprised and excited about the positive impact these simple practices have on the outcomes they work so hard to achieve.

Conversations Worth Having translates evidence-based principles into a practical framework that will enhance your self-awareness, bridge the communication gap, and empower you to shift any conversation into one worth having!

Conversations are the currency of change; they influence every aspect of healthcare delivery. For this reason, we are committed to sharing these practices with the broad spectrum of healthcare professionals. If you have a bias or assumption that communication is a "soft skill" in medicine and therefore should be relegated to someone else on the care team, read this book! Quality communication is a primary tool to care for and heal the current fragmented conditions in healthcare.

Suppressing or ignoring the need for genuine human connection in medicine has come at significant cost for healthcare professionals. Burnout symptoms (exhaustion, depersonalization, and perceived inefficacy) are epidemic. Rampant cynicism and oppositional "othering" impair our interactions with insurance companies, administrative colleagues, and our patients. In response, healthcare professionals are leaving healthcare, through early retirement, career shifts, or death by suicide.

Conversations Worth Having in Healthcare offers two simple communication practices that promise to improve professional satisfaction for those who practice them. Consider how shifting from a narrow "deficit-based" focus to curiosity might relieve burnout and cynicism. How accepting the current reality of the inequities in care delivery systems, while fostering hope and action to tackle these challenges, might create positive change. What might be possible if we pause and tap into the shared humanity of professionals, patients, caregivers, and colleagues? How might pausing and reflection produce dialogue that advances medical care and sustains those who work in healthcare?

As healthcare professionals, we have gifts of knowledge, experience, procedural skills, and training. When applied in the complex context of medical care delivery, we can save patients' lives. None of us do it alone. Physicians, podiatrists, optometrists, PhDs, DNPs, EdDs, dentists, pharmDs, and others with a doctorate degree are all healthcare professionals. So are nurses, insurance analysts, leaders, and managers, housekeeping and food service staff, transport colleagues, behavioral health counselors, therapist wizards (speech, music, physical (PT), occupational (OT), recreational, respiratory and others), technicians (medical, radiology, pharmacy, etc.), assistants (medical, administrative, OT/PT, respiratory, nursing, personal care, etc.), and countless others. The landscape of healthcare delivery is wide and complex; we cannot individually list all of the professionals who serve patients. Know that this book's content is relevant and accessible to each of you. If you are a patient or supporting someone receiving healthcare, you will find the two simple communication practices valuable as well.

There is an old joke that goes, "Why do they call it the **practice** of medicine? With all of that schooling, haven't you figured it out yet?" Our reply, "It's the **practice** of medicine because we are never done learning. We must grow, evolve, unlearn, and apply new knowledge and skills to our caregiving for our entire lives." The two practices you'll learn in this book—generative questions and positive framing—are skills worth learning. Applying them will dramatically increase your effectiveness and joy in your daily interactions. Let us begin!

Elizabeth Warner, MD FACP CPE
warnerwellbeing@gmail.com

Fasiha Haq, Senior Director Global Medical Affairs Education
fasiha@conversationsworthhaving.today

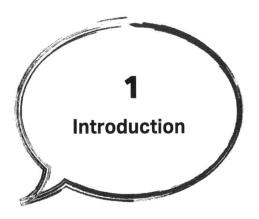

1

Introduction

"Everything happens through conversation."[1]

—*Ron Fry, co-creator of Appreciative Inquiry*

Every conversation you have is moving you in one direction or another. This is especially salient in interactions among healthcare providers, patients, and families. Intentionally fostering conversations worth having turns a potentially mechanistic transaction—treating an illness—into a humanistic interaction—treating the person who has the illness. Effective empathetic communication improves accuracy of diagnosis, adherence to treatment, overall clinical outcomes, and improves healthcare satisfaction for patients and physicians.[2] Unfortunately, miscommunication in healthcare is not isolated.

Studies show that a minority of clinicians ask patients about their health concerns and frequently interrupt before patients get a chance to complete their thoughts.[3] This is a missed opportunity to gather important information. Interruptions increase the likelihood of last-minute concerns being raised and prolonging the visit. Example: "Oh, by the way. I'm having chest pain, but only when I climb stairs."

With intense competing demands on healthcare professionals' attention, it is challenging to be fully present with each patient. They often believe there is not enough time, resulting in a chronic stress response. In reality, studies show if patients are allowed to speak uninterrupted, they finish in about 92 seconds[4], less than two minutes! If healthcare professionals can be fully present and listen to patients' concerns, goals, and perspectives, it improves patients' emotional health, their physiological response, and even reduces pain. For healthcare professionals, this connection results in fewer mistakes, fewer malpractice cases, lower rates of provider stress and burnout,[5] and increased professional satisfaction.[6]

Medical training emphasizes close-ended questions to narrow clinical possibilities to a short list of diagnoses. "Is the pain sharp or dull? Does it hurt when you walk? Does eating make it worse? Have you had this before?" These questions yield important information but miss the patient's story and perspective. Open-ended questions give the patient a chance to provide crucial context. "Describe the pain. What activities make it worse? How long has it been this way? What do you think is going on?" This tells a more complete story than simple isolated facts and is gathered through conversation.

The flagship book, *Conversations Worth Having: Using Appreciative Inquiry to Fuel Productive and Meaningful Engagement*,[7] introduces four types of conversations, a strategy to support deliberate communication, and two simple practices.

What Kind of Conversations Are You Having?

Whether it is our internal dialogue or external interactions with others, being aware of the nature of our conversations is vitally important. With awareness of our words and focus, we can deliberately foster conversations worth having.

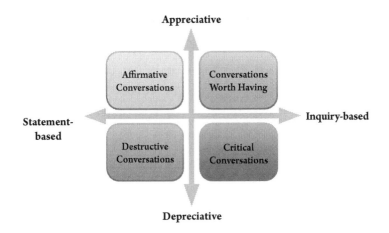

Figure 1.1 The Nature of Our Conversations

Conversations take place along two dimensions: appreciative or depreciative and statements or questions. The result is four types of conversations as shown in Figure 1.1.[8] You will deepen your understanding of the effect of these conversations through examples in chapter 3.

Appreciative Conversations: Above the Line

Conversations above the horizontal line are appreciative: people feel valued and the conversation itself adds value. These interactions have a positive tone and are outcomes-focused. There are two types of appreciative conversations:

1. *Conversations Worth Having.* These interactions add value through inquiry and dialogue.

2. *Affirmative Conversations.* These interactions add value through appreciative comments and statements.

Depreciative Conversations: Below the Line

Conversations below the horizontal line are depreciative: people feel devalued and cannot contribute. Such interactions have a negative tone and direction. There are two types of depreciative conversations:

1. *Critical Conversations.* These interactions devalue people and situations through depreciative questions and transactional interactions.

2. *Destructive Conversations.* These interactions devalue through depreciative comments and statements.

Tone and *direction* are crucial cues to the nature of your conversation. Often just pausing, taking a deep breath, and getting curious about the nature of your conversation is enough to encourage you to ask, *Where am I?* If you're below the line, in a depreciative state, reorient yourself before continuing a conversation. We call this technique *Tuning In.* It's an essential step to intentionally foster conversations worth having. You'll learn more about how to tune in as a healthcare professional in chapter 4.

Let's take a look at two simple practices to support conversations above the line.

Two Simple Practices

Asking generative questions and using positive framing (see Figure 1.2)[9] have been widely and successfully applied in healthcare as well as in families, communities, business, and education all over the world. The conversations from these practices result in increased wellbeing, improved relationships, enhanced goal achievement, innovations, improved patient and employee satisfaction, increased staff retention, and improved financial outcomes.[10] How much of your time inside and outside of work is spent in conversations worth having? How might life change for you and those around you if you deliberately foster conversations worth having? Applying these practices will allow you to turn any conversation—anytime, anywhere—into one worth having.

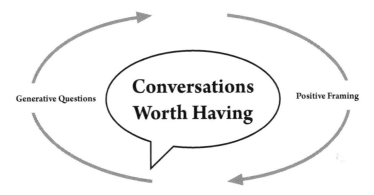

Figure 1.2 Two Simple Practices

Generative Questions

A generative question expands the way people think and the images they hold. In chapter 5, you will read stories illustrating how generative questions bolster patient outcomes and the quality of healthcare professionals' interactions. You'll learn how generative questions add value in diagnostic and treatment conversations. In addition, you'll explore using the practice in common healthcare conversations such as seeking informed consent, understanding goals of care, collaborating with colleagues, and generally supporting better patient outcomes.

The key to asking generative questions is to adopt an attitude of curiosity about people, life, and work. When we are genuinely curious, we ask better questions. When dealing with difficult issues, generative questions make the invisible

visible and bring the background context into the foreground for evaluation and consideration. Such conversations create trust, positive energy, and empower people to move forward in a desired direction.[11] This results in creative problem solving and compelling images for positive action, which is needed to strengthen and improve outcomes in healthcare.

Throughout this book, you'll read stories illustrating the practical and effective use of generative questions. In the appendix, you will find a list of generative questions to support your ongoing practice.

Positive Framing

Rather than focusing on problems and what you don't want to have happen, positive framing focuses on the desired outcomes and what you want to have happen. A positive frame invites people into a future that inspires hope, curiosity, and connection. In chapter 6, you will read stories about how positive framing supports effective conversations.

This practice should not be mistaken for focusing only on the positive; it is not some saccharine misrepresentation of clinical reality. Quite the contrary, this is about dealing with even the toughest issues in a way that increases individual energy and motivation to create positive change. We'll share a technique called *Flipping*[12] to help you, your colleagues, and patients take any issue and create a positive frame. This three-step process is shown in Figure 1.3.[13] The steps are:

- **Name It.** What is the problem, complaint, or the thing you don't want?
- **Flip It.** What is the positive opposite?
- **Frame It.** What is the positive impact if the flip is true; what is the desired outcome?

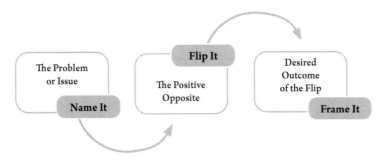

Figure 1.3 The Flipping Technique

In chapter 6, you'll see how negative or problematic frames can be flipped in ways that support shared decision making, empower patients on their healthcare journey, and infuse hope into healthcare interactions.

Appreciative Inquiry: What Gives Life?

Generative questions and positive framing are the foundational practices of Appreciative Inquiry (AI), which is used around the world to foster positive change.[14] The essence of AI is to uncover the best of what is and what can be. It's about discovering what "gives life" to individuals and systems. AI helps healthcare professionals support patients' lives to have meaning and joy, even in the face of illness and crisis.

The Principles Informing Your Conversations

Dr. David Cooperrider identified patterns underlying the research supporting AI.[15] He summarized those patterns in five principles[16] reinforcing just how fateful our conversations are:

1. The Constructionist Principle: *Words create worlds.* What we believe to be true is informed by and evolves through conversation.

2. The Simultaneity Principle: *Inquiry creates*

change. As words are spoken, our mind, body, and emotions react in a split second.

3. The Anticipatory Principle: *We see what we expect to see.* Whatever we anticipate, we are likely to encounter.

4. The Poetic Principle: *There are many aspects to any person, situation, or system.* Our understanding depends upon where we place our attention.

5. The Positive Principle: *Positive image begets positive action begets positive results.* Our questions inspire images, and imagery compels action.

It's Not Magic, It's Science

It's not just "nice" to have conversations worth having, it is essential for healthy relationships, wellness, and productivity. In *Conversations Worth Having: Using Appreciative Inquiry to Fuel Productive and Meaningful Engagement,* Jackie Stavros and Cheri Torres bring together the scientific research behind the two practices. Appreciative Inquiry, neuropsychology, neurophysiology, and positive psychology have all shown that the nature of our conversation is fateful.[17] A conversation that is generative gives people access to greater energy, creativity, self-motivation, and relational capacity. In addition, it fortifies the immune system and enhances resilience.[18] Healthcare needs increased positive energy to drive all the changes needed for selfcare, patient care, and improving the systems we work in. You can experience the energy of conversations by doing the short exercise below.

Experience the Power of Conversation

Take this moment to vividly recall a recent negative conversation you've had with yourself or another person. Notice how that conversation feels in your body. Do you feel a sense of tension or heaviness? Perhaps your heart rate and/or blood pressure increased. If someone was observing, they might have seen your jaw tighten or a distressed expression cross your face.

Pause again, take a deep breath, and let that conversation go. Now, recall an uplifting conversation you've had recently. Use all your senses and notice how that feels in your body. Most people experience a relaxation response that could include your heart rate and blood pressure normalizing. An observer might see your face light up and a smile emerge. Our bodies reflect the power of our conversations. They correlate with distinct biochemical changes, triggering a cascade of emotions, memories, and reactions.

Imbalanced Dialogue

In *Conversations Worth Having*, Jackie and Cheri provide evidence for a necessary ratio of positive to negative interactions to strengthen relationships, find solutions, or achieve desired results. While the studies ranged from 3:1 up to 6:1,[19] they suggest striving for a 4:1 ratio positive to every negative interaction. Engaging in conversations worth having 80% of the time enhances wellbeing and resilience for individuals and fosters a culture of positivity, engagement, and flourishing for families, organizations, and communities.

Putting the Two Practices to Work in Healthcare

We wrote this book for healthcare professionals interacting with patients and their support systems. Imagine using these two practices to learn more about patients, increase trust among your colleagues, patients, and their families, and energize your day. While these two practices are simple, changing behavior is not. It will take practice. This book will show you how.

Though the focus of this book is aimed at transforming healthcare conversations, it has been our experience that these practices have a ripple effect impacting many relationships, including your relationship with yourself.

Let's begin by looking at the significant impact that subtle changes in our conversations can make. We encourage you to learn, apply, and share these practices with your patients, colleagues, and family.

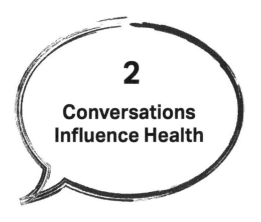

2

**Conversations
Influence Health**

"One good conversation can shift the
direction of change forever."

—*Linda Lambert*

Betty Manolo is sitting upright, ankles crossed, and purse
perched on her knees in a crowded primary care waiting room.
It's been so long since she's seen a doctor. She is worried but
striving to maintain a placid exterior. The waiting room door
opens, and a young man calls out, "Mrs. Manolo?" Betty stands
and quickly crosses the waiting room.

Conner is the medical assistant. He gets her weight and
vital signs, asks what medications she takes, and Betty replies,
"None." Conner pauses, looks down at his computer screen,
and verifies, "Um, you were born 7/19/1955?" She confirms
that she is, indeed, 67 years old, and takes no prescription medications. Conner queries about over the counter meds, vitamins,
and homeopathic remedies. Betty responds, "I have Tylenol for
aches and pains, and I take maybe two pills a month." Conner

asks, "So, what brings you in today?" This is the dreaded question. Betty didn't want to voice her concern once, much less several times during the visit. She gulps, "I can't catch my breath, and it seems to be getting worse." Conner types confidently into his laptop, and upon exiting, breezily offers, "Ok! The doc will be with you shortly!"

Twenty-two minutes later, there is a quick rap upon the door, and she hears, "Mrs. Manolo, may I come in?" Betty affirms the request, and a tall woman in a long white coat enters the room, introducing herself as Dr. Jackson. She shakes Betty's hand, sits on the small rolling stool, and looks up into Betty's face. Dr. Jackson asks what name she prefers and offers her a seat in one of the chairs, off the high perch of the exam table. Betty sinks gratefully into the chair where she rests her feet upon the ground, but sits bolt upright, without leaning against the back.

Dr. Jackson asks, "The notes say that you have shortness of breath? Is that right?" Betty says, "Well, sort of. I am not sure what shortness of breath means, but I get breathless easily. I maintain my home, vacuuming, dusting, cleaning, and such. I find that I have to rest when I am using the hand vacuum on the stairs. I didn't think much of it, until this spring, when I began to prepare my garden beds. I struggled to carry and lift the potting soil, fertilizer, and even had to rest about halfway through mowing the lawn." Betty pauses, embarrassed by speaking so much. She doesn't usually talk freely. In the past, at her husband Louis' doctor visits, she always felt like she was being cross examined. She had to answer the rapid-fire questions shot at her by Louis' doctor with exacting, concise replies. The doctor ended every appointment, hand on doorknob, with, "Louis, she's taking good care of you! Keep it up!" Betty never felt good about the care she gave Louis. She couldn't make him better. He still died.

In her reverie, Betty doesn't hear a question. "I'm sorry, what did you ask?" Dr. Jackson repeats herself, "What are you hoping I can do for you today?" Betty's internal voice screams, "TELL ME I DON'T HAVE CANCER!" On the outside, she maintains her composed face and says, "I just want to be checked out, to be sure that I'm ok. Maybe I'm making too much of this."

Dr. Jackson reassures her that she is wise to come in and is glad to work with Betty to figure out what is going on. She expresses admiration for how active Betty is and inquires more about her home and garden. Betty shares a bit more with each question, and she smiles broadly when asked, "What brings you joy?" Betty beams and leans in to reply, "Oh, I love to garden. It is where I feel closest to heaven and my dear Louis! Whenever I feel down, I just go to the garden. I have kept one forever! That's why I really started to worry when I couldn't do my regular activities without resting. I don't know what I would do without my garden ..." Betty trails off, feeling self-conscious.

Dr. Jackson says, "Thank you so much for sharing! It sounds like your garden really is your happy place! Please take some slow breaths, in and out, while I listen to your lungs." The interview and examination wrap up, and Dr. Jackson sits down to review the computerized medical records.

"Betty, you haven't been in the office for any medical care for almost three years! You MUST be concerned with these current symptoms since you scheduled an appointment." She turns and looks directly into Betty's eyes, "What concerns you most about your breathlessness?" Dr. Jackson seems genuinely curious, and in that space, Betty's defenses drop. Her voice wavers, "I'm worried it's cancer."

Dr. Jackson pauses, carefully forming her next question. "What do you know about cancer that makes you worry?" Betty looks up, startled. She assumes everyone knows she's a widow and that Louis died of lung cancer. Her voice is stronger when she replies, "I KNOW cancer. I watched it eat away at my husband, Louis, until he died two and a half years ago."

The words hang in the air. Dr. Jackson holds the space between them. She takes a deep breath, and acknowledges, "Yes, you DO know cancer intimately. I'm sorry for your loss." After another second or two, the doctor continues, "I would like to ask a few more questions before developing a plan with you. May I?" Betty nodded.

Together, they review more of Betty's history and preventive care records. Dr. Jackson recommends a chest x-ray, which can be done today, and blood work, which Conner can draw. Betty agrees with the plan and feels reassured. When Dr. Jackson leaves, she shakes Betty's hand and says, "I'm glad that you came in today to discuss your symptoms and how you are feeling. We will work together to figure this out. I look forward to our follow up visit in two weeks." Dr. Jackson exits, and Betty thinks, "Funny, I'm looking forward to our next appointment too. I've never had such a nice conversation with a doctor."

Labs and chest x-ray complete, Betty Manolo goes home with a lighter heart. She feels reassured that she has found a doctor who listens deeply, acknowledges her concerns, and develops a plan with her.

Two days later she receives a call from the office. It's Conner. "Your labs all look good, but your chest x-ray suggests we should run some additional tests. Dr. Jackson told me to let you know there is nothing on the x-ray that looks like cancer. She wanted to be sure that I said that so you wouldn't worry. She wants you to do a special breathing test called a Pulmonary Function Test (PFT). I contacted that office to schedule it, and luckily, they had a cancellation for this Friday. Can you make it?" Betty eagerly accepts the appointment, gathers the details, and hangs up with relief. "IT'S NOT CANCER!" She takes a deep breath, smiles, and exhales as if she had been holding her breath for days.

The PFTs show diminished breathing capacity and a CT scan of the chest confirms no cancer but reveals changes in her lungs consistent with emphysema or chronic obstructive pulmonary disease (COPD). At the follow up appointment, Dr. Jackson sits alongside Betty, reviews all the data, and shares the diagnosis.

Betty has a long journey ahead of her to effectively manage this chronic disease. Consider all the healthcare professionals who will be involved in her care: doctors, nurses, respiratory therapists, medical assistants, pharmacists, and durable medical equipment suppliers. Now consider all the responsibilities and time constraints pressuring each of these healthcare professionals. Imagine the different kinds of conversations she is likely to have along her journey. How might those conversations affect her health, wellbeing, and longevity?

Conversations: Above and Below the Line

Words are powerful. They influence the way we hear a story, see another person, and translate a medical interview into the record. Words influence how we see and treat each other. As healthcare professionals, our words are used to communicate our beliefs about a patient's condition, diagnosis, prognosis, and treatment plan. Our conversations move us in either a positive or negative direction; there is no neutral. When conversations move us in a positive direction, they are above the line (appreciative) giving hope, easing fears, and fortifying our immune system. When they move us in a negative direction, they are below the line (depreciative), leaving us anxious and uncertain, stressing the body, and depleting our energy. It is paramount for us to intentionally use our words to connect, uplift, and empower our patients to move above the line. We can do that by having conversations worth having.

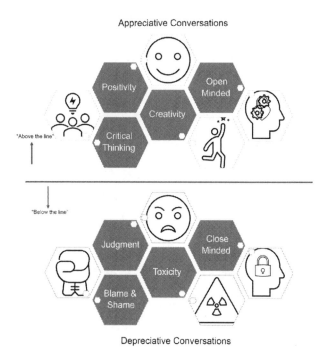

Figure 2.1 Outcomes of Conversations Above and Below the Line

Recall Figure 1.1 from chapter 1. Appreciative conversations are above, and depreciative conversations are below the line. We can sort our interactions in reference to this imaginary horizontal line (see Figure 2.1[20]). When we are below the line, life can be overwhelming, stressful, and unmanageable. We typically feel the need to protect ourselves to survive. This is the world of blame, control, and negative projections (on self and others). When patients come to see us because they have a problem, they are generally below the line. When we are stressed for time or anxious about a diagnosis, we are below the line. Anyone below the line is more likely to foster depreciative conversations, which reinforce everyone's negative experience.

When we are above the line, things in life seem hopeful,

curiosity is activated, and there is potential for creative solutions. When we are above the line, it is easier for us to connect with others, feel empathy, and relate. When our patients engage above the line, it supports their wellbeing, willingness to follow our advice, and healing. When we intentionally foster patient conversations above the line, it uplifts us as well. Above the line, we are more energized to handle our workload. [We encourage you to pause reading and watch a 3-minute video to deepen your understanding of what we mean by "above and below the line." Search YouTube for *Locating Yourself—A Key to Conscious Leadership* https://www.youtube.com/watch?v=fLqzYDZAqCI]

Wired for Protect and Connect

All of us are wired for above the line (attachment, connection, and growth) and below the line (self-protection and survival) interactions. Below the line protection aids in our survival, and above the line connection supports our ability to thrive.

Patients often show up below the line with varying degrees of capacity to shift above the line. The healthcare professional has significant influence in whether they stay there. When healthcare professionals are above the line and present, we can ask generative questions that invite others to move beyond the patterns and adaptive strategies of 'protect' to 'connect'. Then, patients can rediscover what brings them joy and vitality in ways that support wellbeing and healing.

Betty had plenty of reasons for below the line thinking, including the experience of caring for her husband, Louis. Her first conversation with Dr. Jackson invited a healthy doctor-patient relationship built on honesty, caring, and compassion. Betty left the office above the line, in a hopeful space.

Conversations play a vital role in care delivery and are integral in healthcare systems. Informed consent for a procedure occurs through conversation. Explaining a diagnostic work up requires conversation and medical translation. Instructing a patient on how to hold his/her body during an imaging test (e.g., mammogram or CT scan) requires a conversation. Advising on treatment and adherence to a medical treatment plan (myocardial infarction post-care, or hypertension) requires ongoing conversation. Conversation is the currency of change. Medical care is all about change.

We hope the stories in this book informed by the two practices inspire you to have conversations worth having; they are crucial to the wellbeing of patients and those who care for them. Let's begin with understanding the power of conversation.

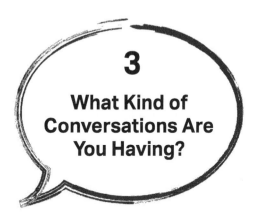

3

What Kind of Conversations Are You Having?

"People will forget what you said, people will forget what you did, but people will never forget how you made them feel."

—*Maya Angelou*

"Mrs. Patel, I have all your test results now. I'm sorry to inform you that you have advanced ovarian cancer throughout your abdomen. I'd like to begin chemotherapy to shrink the tumors in hopes we can operate in the future. Now, given your diabetes and poor kidney function, we can't give you the best drug. We will give you a milder version and assess as we go. I'm sure you have questions. Our nurse, Brenda, will be in shortly to answer them." Dr. Rainier exited the room. Mrs. Patel could barely breathe. Her mind was a flurry of confused questions, "How can I have cancer? I don't smoke, drink, or eat junk food. How did I get this? Could the tests be wrong?"

Her mind raced from one thought to another. She didn't

notice when Brenda entered. "Mrs. Patel? Dr. Rainier is one of the best. You're in great hands. Do you have any questions?" Mrs. Patel was startled by the voice. Tears welled in her eyes as she stammered, "What's…next?"

Just down the hall a very different conversation was taking place. "Ms. Rodriguez, how are you feeling?" said Dr. Zeta, a cardiologist. "I want to thank you for your patience."

Dr. Zeta looked up at those sitting around the room. "Is this your family? Who's here?" Family members introduced themselves. He approached each person, shook hands, repeating each person's name, "Hi! I'm Dr. Zeta. It's a pleasure to meet you."

Then, with calm demeanor and patience, Dr. Zeta began to explain the test results, "Your EKG shows electricity flowing through your heart. This area raises concern that your heart muscle is not getting the oxygen that it needs. Does that make sense to you, Ms. Rodriguez?" He asked.

She nodded and added, "Is that why I've been lightheaded and tired when I climb stairs?" "Possibly," he responded. "We have some options for treating this. I would like to discuss these with you. Would you like your family to stay for this conversation?" She nodded again. He looked at her family and smiled, "You have a lot of people who love and care about you. You are so lucky." Ms. Rodriguez replied with a big grin, "Yes, I am. I thank God every day!"

In these two stories, both patients have serious, life-threatening diagnoses. Both physicians are knowledgeable and competent. Each patient's experience was different due to the kind of conversation they had about the diagnosis. One doctor was mechanistic, focusing on the disease, and the other humanistic, focusing on the person. The healthcare professional's approach has a significant effect on patients. Multiple studies show that verbal and non-verbal communication that acknowledges and validates patient emotions, circumstances, and perspectives results in meaningful connections which foster trusting partnerships.[21] Let's take a look at the nature of these two conversations.

The Nature of Our Conversations

As you learned in chapter 1, the conversations we have fall across two dimensions and reflect whether people's interactions are above the line (appreciative) or below the line (depreciative). Refer back to Figure 1.1. In the first story above, Dr. Rainier fostered a depreciative conversation, triggering panic and speechlessness within Mrs. Patel. In the second story, Dr. Zeta initiated an appreciative conversation with Ms. Rodriguez and her family, resulting in shared understanding about the diagnosis.

Appreciative conversations can occur in any situation. Even bad news can be delivered in a way that supports connection, wellbeing, and health. In medical settings, these conversations impact the quality, length, and trajectory of a patient's life.[22] Let's look at common interactions in the four conversation quadrants: destructive, critical, affirmative, and conversations worth having, and consider how the scenarios above reflect the power of a conversation in influencing patient interactions and medical care.

Depreciative Conversations

Recall that depreciative conversations can be destructive, critical, or a blend of both. Any healthcare professional who feels pressured by time and dueling priorities is more likely to engage in matter-of-fact and direct communication. These conversations can have detrimental consequences, regardless of the healthcare professional's intent. Here are a few examples of depreciative conversations.

Destructive Conversations

"I'm not going into the hospital." Anna's mother was adamant. "Don't be so silly," chided Anna. "The doctor said you need to be checked in for a series of tests while they monitor your heart. Do you want to pack your bag or shall I?" Her mother exploded, "I am not going, and you can't make me. I want to die at home!" "You're being ridiculous, Mom. You're not going to die." Anna was irritated. She began to pack a bag. Her mother pushed the bag to the floor.

This depreciative conversation is destructive since it's all statement based. They are talking past one another, not with one another. How might this interaction have shifted if Anna asked, "Why are you so adamant about not going to the hospital?" Anna would have learned that her mom's father believed that people go into hospitals and never come out. His strong voice in her head had her focusing on all the people she'd known that had checked into the hospital and died there. If Anna had been aware of this, she could have shifted the conversation, helping her mom remember her many friends who had successfully entered and discharged from the hospital, and were still alive and well.

Critical Conversations

The nurse manager looked stern as she motioned for the certified nursing assistant, Franklin, to step into her office. Before he could close the door, the manager barked, "What were you thinking when you told the patient what was in his chart? Didn't they teach you anything in orientation?" Franklin meekly replied, "I was trying to be helpful because the patient was really stressed. His blood pressure was up, and his heart rate was…" The manager cut him off, asking critically, "and what are you supposed to do if you are worried about a patient's condition?"

Franklin defended, "I tried to get a nurse to come in, but..."
Again, the manager interrupted, "I don't want excuses. Do that again, and you won't be working here!"

This is a critical conversation: the supervisor's questions devalue Franklin. The nurse manager is not really interested in learning about the situation nor Franklin's reasoning. The questions are laden with assumptions and judgment. If she had been genuinely curious, she might have asked, "How did you come to give this patient information from his chart? Share your thinking with me." She would have learned a lot. Franklin noticed the patient's emotional distress, and that his pulse was 120. He tried to get a nurse, per protocol, but the nurse was occupied at the far end of the hall. With the patient's heart condition, Franklin was worried he might have a heart attack or stroke. Franklin reassured and calmed the patient by reporting that his labs were normal, but the medical team would review them in detail. The nurse manager and Franklin might then have branched into a conversation about calming strategies for patients and how to connect with a nurse during a busy shift. Each of these could have been conversations worth having.

Recall Dr. Rainier and Mrs. Patel. Dr. Rainier is highly qualified, and while not intentionally critical, her word choice and the way she delivers her diagnosis resulted in a depreciative interaction. Dr. Rainier delivered information without connecting to her patient in any way. As a result, Mrs. Patel felt overwhelmed, confused, and very scared. The neurophysiological response to these emotions involves the release of cortisol, norepinephrine, testosterone, and other stress hormones and neurotransmitters that amplify her emotional state. This makes it impossible for Mrs. Patel to form any clear or thoughtful questions for nurse Brenda to answer.

When people are not intentional in their healthcare conversations, they can often end up in depreciative interactions. Consider the intake nurse who doesn't make eye contact but keeps asking terse questions. When the answers don't come, she simply repeats the question louder. The son or daughter who is frustrated that their parent refuses to take their medication; chastising them again and again leaving the parent shamed and even more confused. The irritated patient barking demands at the care provider, who bites their tongue and responds by providing the minimum care.

Depreciative conversations don't help patients feel better or recover faster. They create cold, sterile, and even hostile environments, which weaken a patient's capacity for wellbeing and healing. They are detrimental to every human in these interactions—healthcare professionals, patients, and their family members and loved ones.[23]

Appreciative Conversations

In contrast, appreciative conversations are enlivening. These take the form of affirmative conversations and conversations worth having. Much of the time, these two kinds of conversation blend in ways that add value and support health and wellbeing.

Dr. Zeta's conversation was appreciative. Even though Ms. Rodriguez has a significant heart condition, he was able to engage in a conversation with her in ways that generated connection, positive emotions, and hope. The neurotransmitters and hormones that correlate with such conversations support the potential for health and healing: oxytocin, serotonin, endorphins, and dopamine.[24]

Dr. Zeta took the time to blend affirmative statements with generative. When he said, "Thanks for your patience. You have a lot of people who love and care about you," he was fostering an affirmative conversation. He engaged in a conversation worth having when he shared information and asked questions to connect with the patient and her entire family. There are many opportunities in healthcare for both affirmative conversations and conversations worth having. Here are a few examples.

Affirmative Conversations

Dr. Sinclair smiles while sharing recent test results with Bill. "Nice work, Bill. Clearly, you've been taking the medication. Your blood sugar is right where we want it. And I can see you've been watching your diet and exercising. You're doing great!"

In the physical therapy room, son John looks at his father and smiles. "Papa," he said, "you're doing great with those exercises the doctor gave you. Just look how much better you move already! I know it's been hard; I'm so proud of you."

In the next building over, Tom, the surgical nurse, and Dr. VanLuven are having an affirmative conversation with few words. Tom anticipated the surgeon's every need, making sure she had the right instrument with precise timing. In Tom's mind, they were a team, working to save this patient. Exhausted after three hours of emergency surgery, Dr. VanLuven turned to Tom saying, "Thank you so much, Tom. What a pleasure it is to work with you, we were really in sync! I wish every surgical team I had in the operating room felt like that!"

Affirmative conversations have an appreciative tone that supports positive emotions and strengthens relationships; however, without inquiry, these conversations do not deepen shared knowledge, spark creative thinking, or encourage collaborative action. Any of these conversations can easily transition into a conversation worth having, simply by asking generative questions.

Conversations Worth Having

Dr. Sinclair continues, **"What's your secret, Bill? What's made you successful in remembering to take your meds, exercise, and eat healthy?"** Bill shares that he'd used a process of making small changes and then adding to it over time that he'd learned from a TEDx Talk by BJ Fogg, called *Forget Big Change, Start with a Tiny Habit*.[25] He matched taking his meds with a habit he already had, brushing his teeth, and he grew his habit of exercising and pairing it with going to use the bathroom. Bill chuckles over how he expects to get more and more exercise as he gets older! Bill leaves his 15-minute visit feeling great and encouraged to do more. Dr. Sinclair learned techniques he can offer other patients. It was definitely a conversation worth having.

John's dad beams. John continues, "How'd you motivate yourself? With mama gone, I was worried about your recovery." His father replies, "John, your mama was not the only person who's important to me. You and your sisters are important, and your kids. I want to be able to play with 'em and watch 'em grow up." John takes the opportunity to share his concerns, "Papa, I want that too. And I'm worried that the way you eat is going to prevent that. You've done so well moving around, can we talk about making just a few diet changes?" His dad looks skeptical. John asks, "What foods did the doctor say were unhealthy?" "He said sugar was the worst for me, but I'm not willing to give up my sweets!" John replies, **"What if we make desserts that are sweet, but don't have any sugar in them?** Would you be willing to try?" John's dad asks, "How ya gonna do that?" It turns into a conversation worth having.

Tom thanks Dr. VanLuven and asks, "I enjoyed working with you as well. I would love for every surgery to flow like that one. What do you think about the new teamwork effort the administration is making?" The doctor gives the response Tom anticipates, "If I could have people like you on my team every time, I think it would be great. But we know that's not the case." Tom follows up, "But, what if we could? I don't do anything other nurses couldn't do if they were trained and had the opportunity." The doctor layers on more praise. "I appreciate the compliments a lot," he said, "and I would love to explore what you found so helpful. Can you tell me what I did that made me such a valuable team player?" Dr. VanLuven outlines several behaviors she appreciated in surgery, behaviors that helped her remain attentive to the patient. Tom nods and replies, **"What if we find out what every surgery team member does that contributes to team excellence and patient care, and design training based on that information?"** By the time their conversation is over, the surgeon is open to building this high-performing team concept. This is a conversation worth having.

Appreciative conversations support everyone in the conversation, not just patients. Ultimately, patients need to have conversations above the line. Recall that a 4:1 ratio of positive to negative interactions strengthens relationships and supports desired outcomes. This means we must strive for a lot more positive interactions in our daily conversations.

Fostering Conversations Above the Line

Fostering conversations above the line sounds simple, but it's not always easy. It requires us to tune in to ourselves: our emotional landscape, physical state, and mindset. We refer to this as the body-mindset. It requires conscious awareness, deliberate choice, and effort to foster appreciative conversations. It is even more challenging to stay above the line when feeling time-pressured, energy lagging, or when reacting to negative energy from others in the room.

Take for example, Mr. Bee, recovering from a complex femur fracture in a skilled nursing facility. He is tired of being in constant pain and frustrated by his dependence on the staff. He feels like a child, and he hates that. His body-mindset is way below the line. When staff or family come to his room, they are met with that negative energy, and his comments emerge from that deeply negative space. If staff entering his room don't raise their awareness about what's influencing Mr. Bee's actions, it is likely they too will be pulled below the line. This will likely result in a depreciative conversation.

When healthcare professionals and family members raise their awareness, they can be intentional about their interactions. In the next chapter, we share a simple strategy to help anyone prime themselves for a conversation worth having—anytime and in any situation. We call this strategy *tuning in*.

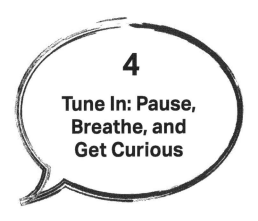

4

**Tune In: Pause,
Breathe, and
Get Curious**

"When you press the pause button on a machine, it stops.
But when you press the pause button on
human beings, they start."

—*Dov Seidman*

Paul had been suffering from stomach pains for almost four months when he showed up at the doctor's office in September. Paul had a history of childhood cancer and was concerned the pain heralded the cancer's return. Dr. Sharp did his best to reassure Paul. "I'm sure it's nothing," he said, "let's start you on something to reduce stomach acid. You'll feel better in a few days."

At his 6-week follow up visit, Paul's symptoms persisted, and he repeated his concerns. "Doctor, I'm worried this could be some sort of new cancer or related to my previous cancer." Dr. Sharp calmly replied, "Let's not jump to a worst-case scenario.

Let's take this one step at a time. I want you to double up on the medication, and then we can re-evaluate in a few weeks."

The medication did not help; symptoms grew worse. In late April, Paul and his wife, Jackie, were convinced that something was seriously wrong, but the doctor insisted that it was probably gastrointestinal reflux. "We just need to find the right medication or medication level." After six weeks on another medicine, Paul's wife stepped in, "This isn't working. This isn't good enough." They could see Dr. Sharp grow irritated with her authoritative tone. "It is highly unlikely that it is cancer," he scolded. "We don't need to make this into something it's not. But if it makes you feel better, I can order an abdominal ultrasound."

Paul waited anxiously for the results of the test. When the call came, it was Dr. Sharp himself on the phone, "The results aren't good. The scan shows numerous masses in your abdomen that look quite concerning. I want to do some more tests immediately." Paul reacted, "But you said it was stomach acid." "I never said that," defended Dr. Sharp. "I said it *could* be stomach acid, but given your history and the test results…" "So, it's cancer then?" Paul interrupted. "I didn't say that," the doctor said with an edge in his voice.

Paul's fourth and final visit in June turned contentious. Paul's eyes and expression didn't hide his anxiety and anger; how could the doctor have missed 15 tumors? Dr. Sharp's calm, reassuring demeanor was gone. He seemed nervous, cautious, and carefully considering every word before he said it. "We need to get a biopsy for confirmation, so I'm going to refer you to a specialist. From now on, I think it's best if you collaborate with the oncologist. If you need any more information from my office, please contact my office manager." Dr. Sharp strode towards the door, looked back one last time and said, "I did everything that reasonably could have been expected of me. No one could have foreseen this unfortunate turn of events."

Nine months after his initial visit, Paul was diagnosed with an aggressive stage four lymphoma. Imagine the difference that might have occurred if, on that first visit, Dr. Sharp had listened closely to Paul, considered his perspective and ideas, and widened his differential diagnosis and workup. How might tumor growth and staging have been different if Paul had been diagnosed in the fall? They had four conversations, over several months and none of them were worth having.

No one intentionally chooses to have a depreciative conversation. Such interactions happen when we engage without awareness. We're almost always in dialogue, with ourselves or others, and most of the time what's driving our conversations is unconscious. Let's take a look at what pulls conversations below the line.

What Pulls Us Below the Line

Much of the time, we engage in conversation unaware of the influences that drive us above or below the line. Three of these factors are worth further exploration: the invisible ego, the situational context, and the larger culture.

1. The Invisible Ego

The ego is the part of the mind that mediates between the conscious and the unconscious and is responsible for reality testing and a sense of personal identity.[26] Whenever our personal identity or sense of belonging is threatened, our nervous system reacts to protect the ego. This can be an effective response when we are physically threatened, but most of the time, it's ineffective to have conversations from a defensive stance. When we're below the line in a heightened state of protection, our body clues us in: sweaty palms, racing heart, shallow breathing, fuzzy thinking, heat waves, tingling, rising blood pressure, and increasing incoherence in our heart and nervous system.

31

This correlates with big emotions like anger, panic, fear, and overwhelm. Other times, the ego's response to protect is more subtle, without the palpable emotions, but still obstructing authentic interactions.

Consider this example: Dr. Mercer recently graduated from medical school and is now an intern at a prestigious hospital. She fears she doesn't have much to offer. She holds back from contributing during rounds, even when her ideas would add value. She avoids seeking support from others for fear of being judged as inexperienced or ignorant. Dr. Henson, also a first-year intern, has similar insecurities. He compensates by spending his evenings researching new and experimental approaches and then overly sharing what he's read during rounds, even when the information is not relevant to the current patient. He frequently retells his "success stories" to other interns to affirm his competence.

Can you spot the subtle protect strategies each of these interns is using? For their growth and wellbeing, the health and safety of their patients, and to genuinely engage with their colleagues, they need to shift above the line to connect. It can be challenging for all humans to raise our awareness of the subtle protective strategies we use to keep our egos safe.

What forms of protect might have played a role in Dr. Sharp's responses to Paul, especially in subsequent appointments? Dr. Sharp is closed to considering alternative diagnoses and offers simple solutions following standard protocols. When Paul's symptoms get worse, Dr. Sharp doubles down on his diagnosis, getting impatient and defensive. His invisible ego was driving his external behavior, subconsciously perceiving Paul's persistent symptoms as a challenge to his identity as a physician. Six months into the process, everyone involved is below the line, engaged in depreciative conversations.

Healthcare professionals are under a lot of pressure to have answers, to "fix" what's wrong with certainty and speed.

Signs We're Protecting Our Ego	
Perfectionism/trying to get it right	Sarcasm, shaming
Proving that you are good enough	Having a rigid agenda
Trying to control the situation	Addictive patterns
Not engaging/shutting down	Judging, blaming
Passive/aggressive behavior	Defensiveness

It's a challenge to stay open to "not knowing" under those circumstances. Your nervous system reacts to protect you from feelings of inadequacy, shame, guilt, fear, anxiety, incompetence, and uncertainty. It's subtle, until it's not. As a physician, nurse extern, family member, or patient, when you feel yourself getting irritated, defensive, resentful, or submissive, that is your ego.

For patients and families, medical authority can be intimidating. Typically, when self-confident and outspoken individuals grow silent and passive, their ego has driven them into protect and pulled them below the line. Patients often think, "Doctors are the experts. Who am I to question them?" This deferential thinking results in a missed opportunity for a conversation worth having.

2. Situational Context: The Healthcare System

There are significant financial pressures to deliver healthcare services efficiently. Healthcare professionals are encouraged to quickly move from diagnosis to most effective treatment, implemented in the most efficient way. This allows the healthcare professional to see more patients, with the praiseworthy goal of seeking to help the greatest number of people. Other pressures in fee-for-service environments drive professionals to ensure the organization gets reimbursed for services provided and stays within departmental budgets.

These incentives are sometimes at odds with each other and with the patient. Payment for most healthcare services in America is biased towards activity, including lab tests, imaging studies, consultations, medications, procedures, and surgeries. Diagnostic strategies are focused on identifying problems, and the work is focused on treating symptoms and curing diseases.

Healthcare professionals use objective measures like history and physical exam, lab tests, imaging studies, and algorithms to narrow a long list of possible conditions, to the most likely diagnosis to work up and treat. Isolating problems can inadvertently lead healthcare professionals to a default mode of transactional interactions, focusing on the symptoms (sore throat) or organ system (respiratory) versus the complex human patient bearing the physical problem. The patient often holds the key to the disease and their health. It is unlocked through their story.

When healthcare professionals are aware of the situational context of productivity-based healthcare incentives, they can intentionally choose their words and behavior. With awareness, they can foster conversations that allow them to hear the patient's story, stay open and curious, and seek to understand the patient's perspective. While this approach may seem less efficient, the data suggests it is both effective and efficient to gather the patient's story.

"The good physician treats the disease; the great physician treats the patient with the disease."
—*William Osler*

A 2019 study published in the *Journal of General Internal Medicine* found that on average, patients get about 11 seconds to explain the reasons for their visit before they are interrupted by their doctors and that only one in three doctors provides their patients with adequate opportunity to describe their situation.[27] To hear the patient's story, we must actively listen and allow them 90-120 seconds to relate their concern. This time offered up front is often repaid in hours saved through additional testing, return visits, misdiagnosis, and wasted treatment time. Actively listening to the patient yields more effective treatment strategies for supporting the patient's recovery and healing, and it provides the therapeutic benefit of interpersonal connection.[28]

3. Culture

The culture in which we are immersed shapes our beliefs about what is and isn't acceptable, how we should and should not behave, who belongs and who doesn't, what is of value and what is not. Our worldview provides us with a set of assumptions, which filter how we perceive others, how we understand what they tell us, and how we engage in conversation with them. Being unaware of these influences can prime us for depreciative interactions. For example, Dr. Burk saw an overweight, 72-year-old woman in need of shoulder surgery. His version of the "average overweight 72-year-old woman" was sedentary; when he reassured her that she'd be able to garden again after surgery, he was taken aback when she asked, "But will I be able to mountain bike and kayak again?"

The dominant culture in any country influences what is seen as "normal". Healthcare professionals in the dominant culture may default to their experience, creating dangerous blind spots. Marginalized groups of patients and healthcare professionals experience exclusion, judgment, dismissal, misunderstanding, misdiagnosis, or mistreatment as a result. One way through this cultural bias is to practice awareness, stay open minded, and engage in conversations worth having.

As living systems, humans are complex and ever-changing. We are designed to evolve in response to the world around us. As healthcare professionals, it is valuable to approach each patient with a growth mindset.[29] The Zen Buddhist philosophy refers to this as a beginner's *mind*, which reflects an attitude of openness and a lack of preconceptions. Cultivating our beginner's mind invites us to make room for discovery and new knowledge to emerge from a patient's story. Connecting with the patient in this way augments our knowledge, experience, and wisdom.

Seasoned professionals who believe they have "seen it all" are at greater risk for falling into the cognitive fallacy of pattern recognition,[30] and thus prematurely narrowing their inquiry to fit the pattern they expect to see in the patient's symptoms. This likely played a part in Dr. Sharp's conclusion that Paul's symptoms were due to acid reflux.

These three primary influences condition us emotionally and mentally for conversations. To be deliberate with your words, you need to expand your awareness in the present moment, consider the influences you are experiencing, and then consciously choose to foster conversations that are in the best interest of the patient. Here's how Michael did this for his mom.

Michael's mom was hospitalized 1,200 miles away. Each day when he spoke to her, she sounded less coherent. His brother was at her side, "The doctors are doing everything they can. I've called all the relatives. You need to get here fast. She's dying!" Michael arrived the next day and greeted his mom who was groggy and mumbling incoherently. He took a few deep breaths, and then asked to review her chart. She was on nine different medications. He asked the nurses about each drug, they explained their use, but the nurses didn't know about any drug interactions. If she was dying, he wondered, why did she need all these medications? He reviewed the list with his old college roommate, now a hospital pharmacist in Cincinnati. His friend told him that three of the medicines were not indicated for someone with a shortened life expectancy, two of the pills commonly caused muscle pain and sedation, and the frequency of her pain medication dosing could be contributing to her incoherence.

Michael was his mom's designated healthcare power of attorney, and he knew that she wanted to be alert, if possible, in her dying days. He waited for each doctor to round. He shared what he'd learned about her meds and inspired conversations worth having with two of the doctors. Each thanked him for being conscientious and emphasizing what she valued in her care. They discontinued two of the medications and lowered the dosage of two others. The third physician, however, was furious, "Who are you again? I am her doctor!" Michael reached for his mom's hand and gave it a gentle squeeze. He calmly replied, "I am her son. I am telling you that she does not want to be this 'out of it.' She wants to be alert and able to interact with us, even if she's in some pain. From what I've heard from my brother, it's not clear that she IS in pain. Can we reduce the pain medicine and see how she does?" The doctor turned abruptly and left, telling the nurse to stop the pain medication, "Do whatever he says," jerking his thumb at Michael, "He seems to know what's best."

The next morning his mom was more alert, and her speech made more sense. She could ask the nurses for pain medication if needed. Relatives arrived and the room was filled with laughter and the retelling of family memories. She seemed energized by her surrounding family. She transferred home with pain and anxiety medications in case she was suffering. Four days later, she slept throughout the day, taking only sips of water. She opened her eyes when hearing her sons' voices, smiled dreamily, and closed her lids. She died peacefully a few days later. Her final days were full of life.

When you find yourself below the line, remind yourself that wellbeing is more than just physical health. It includes the whole person, their relationships, and their values. Regardless of whether you are a healthcare professional, family member, patient, or friend—give yourself permission to suspend what you think so that you can listen deeply to others and entertain other possibilities. Set your ego aside, be open and curious with whatever is unfolding in the moment. To achieve this, we offer our technique to tune in: *pause, breathe, and get curious.*

Tuning In: Pause, Breathe, and Get Curious

It's easy to have conversations worth having when you're above the line, primed for connection. But what do you do when you're below the line, in protect, with your system on high alert, stressed, and protecting the ego? How can you enhance your capacity for awareness and develop your ability to intentionally foster a conversation worth having?

Tune In

Tuning in and staying tuned in is a strategy that supports intentionality. To tune in, we recommend the technique: pause, breathe, and get curious. It begins with being mindful.

Tuning in is about knowing where you are—above or below the line—and getting curious about where others are. Take time throughout your day to notice your body-mindset[31] and whether you are primed for appreciative or depreciative conversations. Ask yourself: **What am I thinking? What's going on in my body? What am I feeling? Am I feeling rushed, hungry, or content?** Instead of passing judgment on your cur-

> **Practice Tuning In**
>
> Take a moment, pause, take a deep breath, and ask yourself, *Where Am I?* Notice your internal conversation. Don't try and change a thing, just notice.

rent state, just notice it, take a deep breath, and continue with whatever you were doing.

The more you practice tuning in, the more attuned you will become. This alone has the potential to increase your capacity to deliberately foster conversations worth having. However, it may not be enough when you go below the line in the midst of a conversation or react to a specific event. To build your capacity for tuning in during conversations and when you are triggered, we encourage you to pause, breathe, and get curious.

Pause, Breathe, and Get Curious

We typically don't pay attention to our body or our mindset; yet they influence every moment of our day. In any interaction, practicing tuning in makes it easier for you to **PAUSE** before responding, especially when you're in a depreciative conversation.

Pause long enough to intentionally **BREATHE**, inhaling deeply and exhaling slightly longer. This kind of breathing stimulates the parasympathetic nervous system, signaling the body that it's safe to relax.[32] Andrew Huberman's research affirms "the reason a breath practice is so powerful is that it's a bridge between our unconscious, reflexive states and our conscious, deliberate state."[33]

In the space created by this breath, **GET CURIOUS!** Curiosity is a positive emotion;[34] it helps you access your emotional intelligence, creativity, and higher order thinking. You can get curious about yourself by asking generative questions such as:

- **What's really going on here?**
- **What assumptions am I making?**
- **What role is my ego playing in this situation?**
- **How might my action(s) be influenced by hidden biases?**

- **What might I be missing?**
- **What else is going on for me that might be influencing this encounter?**
- **What don't I know?**

You can also get curious about the other person:

- **What different perspective might they have that's important?**
- **What else might be going on for them?**
- **What do they value in this situation?**
- **What motivates them?**
- **What outcome are they hoping for?**

Compassionate Self-Talk*

If you find it difficult to raise your awareness without immediate self-judgment, practice what Dr. Kristen Neff refers to as compassionate self-talk. Dr. Neff's definition of self-compassion includes: 1. Kind self-talk, 2. Mindfulness, 3. Shared humanity. Examples of compassionate self-talk are: "I am enough. It is going to be OK. I am doing the best I can. This is hard for other people too. I can hold space for all feelings, not just the positive ones. I am allowed to make mistakes, all humans do! Today, I will treat myself with kindness. Like any human being, I have strengths and weaknesses." What examples can you generate to turn judgmental thoughts into compassionate self-talk?

*https://self-compassion.org/category/exercises/#exercises

Teaching Patients to Tune In

Regardless of whether patients are above or below the line, tuning in will help them become more aware of their body-mindset and hence better able to support their care and healing process. Patients are often in varying degrees of protect, especially if they have a serious condition. For example, a patient might be dealing with fear, anxiety, shame, rumination, addictive patterns, anger, or blame. They may have researched statistical outcomes, fueling their concerns about what might happen. They may have been in an accident, been given a terrifying diagnosis, or be struggling with some form of dementia.

> **Try this Exercise from Huberman**
>
> "When you inhale, realize that you are literally taking control of your brain and mind. When you exhale, allow that ability to take hold in positive ways. Intentional breathing reminds us that we are in control of our inner state at the most fundamental level. And you can grab ahold of that sense of control anytime stress hits or when you simply want to appreciate a moment and be more present."*
>
> *Dr. Andrew Huberman, Neuroscientist & Head of Madefor Advisory Board
> Excerpt taken from Madefor's Member communications. (www.getmadefor.com)

Whatever thoughts and feelings are sending them below the line, tuning in can help. In the moment, you can literally walk them through tuning in. Calmly invite them to pause and breathe. Take a deep breath yourself as you invite them to breathe deeply. While you breathe with them, invite them to take their time on the exhale. You can help them get curious about their thoughts and feelings and connect with them when they respond.

For example, ask, "**What's happening for you right now? What are you feeling?**" Listen to their responses and reply empathetically. They might tell you they are really frightened about surgery. Instead of trying to fix their feelings, reply, "That's understandable. **What specific concerns do you have?**" As they relay their concerns, you can respond to each one with calm and reassurance. In just a short amount of time, you're likely to see signs that they are shifting above the line: relaxation, deeper breathing, more positive facial expressions, and curiosity about what you are saying or their condition. These signal a much better neurophysiological space for medical care.

Whatever your relationship to a patient, one of the most supportive things you can do is to help them tune in and get above the line.

Listening and Tuning In with a Patient

After falling and injuring her left arm, Mrs. Wong was brought to the orthopedist's office by her daughter, Meili. The ortho technician told Meili to stay in the waiting room. Mrs. Wong flushed, and her heart pounded upon hearing this, giving Meili a worried glance. Meili looked back reassuringly. Mrs. Wong was escorted into an x-ray room for a series of x-rays on both shoulders. Mrs. Wong protested, stating that only one arm was injured. The tech replied, "It's just standard with patients your age. The doctor wants to compare both shoulders." Mrs. Wong was taken to an exam room where her daughter joined her.

Dr. Gray walked in looking at the x-rays on his laptop, "I understand you're experiencing pain in your left shoulder and arm, correct?" Mrs. Wong nodded. "You've lost much of the cushion in your shoulder joints on both sides, and you have significant bone spurs, here and here. You definitely have arthritis," showing them the x-rays. He observed her shoulder range of motion, and Mrs. Wong winced as she raised her arms out to the sides. "Well, you don't need surgery. I can administer a cortisone shot, which should reduce your pain and help your range of motion. I've done a ton of these injections. I'll numb you up. You won't feel a thing. Given what I see in the x-rays, I recommend we treat both shoulders. How does that sound?" She wordlessly nodded.

Dr. Gray exited the room to prepare for the procedure. Mrs. Wong then expressed her concern. "Mom," Meili replied, "You ordinarily speak right up. **What's going on for you right now?**" Mrs. Wong shared that she felt powerless. "He spoke with such authority and experience. I didn't feel like I could say anything.

He is the doctor." Meili paused and said, "Mom, take a deep breath with me, hold it in a sec, and let it out slowly. Good! Now take another." Her mom's face relaxed slightly and Meili asked, **"Now, what would you like the doctor to know?"**

When Dr. Gray returned, Meili made room for her mom to speak. Dr. Gray put the procedure tray down and listened. Mrs. Wong shared, "Dr. Gray, I've known for years that my shoulders have arthritis. I recently fell and injured my left arm. It hurts in a different way. I can move my arms well but raising my left arm out to the side hurts a lot. I am afraid to use it. I feel like it will give out on me. I am worried because this is definitely different from my chronic arthritis pain."

Dr. Gray asked some different questions with this information. **"Walk me through the fall again. What happened? How have the symptoms evolved since the fall?"** Then, Dr. Gray paused, took a deep breath, and smiled at Mrs. Wong, **"What activities do you love to do that require your shoulders?"** he asked. They were now having a conversation worth having. When they were done, Dr. Gray replied, "I think we should get an MRI of that shoulder to look at the soft tissues, which are not well visualized in the x-rays. **How does that sound to you?"**

Anyone in a conversation can tune in and help others tune in if needed. This simple strategy helps healthcare conversations turn from rote and reactive to intentional and generative. Notice the question Meili asked her mom, **"What would you like the doctor to know?"** This is a generative question. Mrs. Wong's answer to Meili's question gave Dr. Gray more information, which changed his thinking about diagnosis and treatment options. This is the nature of generative questions.

In the next chapter, we'll explore generative questions in more detail.

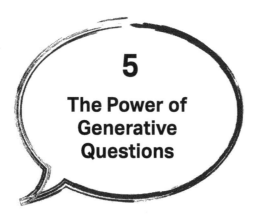

5
The Power of Generative Questions

"Curiosity is more important than knowledge."

—Albert Einstein

Healthcare professionals may consider themselves experts at asking questions of patients. These questions tend to be close-ended and problem-focused, honing in on the patient's presenting complaint. This may narrow the focus too soon, leaving related information and crucial patient-specific context of the medical issue unexplored. Open-ended, generative questions provide more insight into the patient's world. This includes underlying emotions and how they shape the encounter, what outcomes the patient hopes for, and how the patient makes decisions. Such information can greatly enhance the medical care of the patient and the human connection between the healthcare professional and patient.

The type of questions asked are fateful because the interaction is shaped and directed the moment the question is uttered.[35] Beyond a healthcare context, asking generative questions in conversations will improve your chances to better understand others and build genuine connection with them.

The Power of Generative Questions

We can cultivate genuine curiosity when we are tuned in, present, listening, and adopting a growth mindset (or beginner's mind) about the patient's concerns. Generative questions are a natural response to such curiosity. If our attitude embraces such thoughts as, **"What don't I know? What might I be missing?"** without self-judgment, we can ask patients questions that might expand our knowledge and awareness. Generative questions allow us to do all of that in ways that benefit everyone involved.

There are four characteristics of generative questions that inspire connection, ignite hope, and raise awareness. They are open-ended, inviting description, and exploration. They seek depth over brevity, eliciting stories, thoughts, and emotions. They embrace what is, without judgment or agenda. They unlock possibility, tapping into imagination, potential, and opportunity.

Most generative questions result in the following four outcomes. They make the invisible visible, create shared understanding, generate new knowledge, and inspire possibilities.

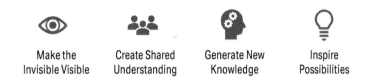

| Make the Invisible Visible | Create Shared Understanding | Generate New Knowledge | Inspire Possibilities |

Figure 5.1 Outcomes from Generative Conversations

Make the Invisible Visible

When body language, tone, and pitch do not match the words someone is saying, there's a need to make what is invisible visible. Incongruence suggests unspoken or unconscious thoughts and feelings are present. A generative question can open this up (see Figure 5.1[36]). Ask yourself:

- **What am I aware of that's unclear: an expression, a tone, a statement, or an intuition?**
- **Is there incongruence between what the person is saying and other signals I am reading (body language, tone, pitch, facial expression, patterns)?**
- **What unspoken assumptions, beliefs, or cultural norms may be influencing my actions or theirs?**

Then, instead of guessing, ask the other person a question that helps make the invisible visible.

- **What concerns and questions do you have?**
- **What's going on for you right now?**
- **What are your thoughts?**
- **What led you to that conclusion?**
- **What informed your decision?**

Create Shared Understanding

Creating shared understanding—whether about the past, present, or future—creates a solid foundation for next steps. Understanding another person's experience or perspective and using empathy builds trust. When healthcare professionals are transparent about their experience or perspective regarding a patient situation, trust is strengthened. When patients thoroughly understand the diagnosis, treatment options, and care protocols, they can more easily move forward with the healthcare team. If you find yourself wondering about something, whether with a patient or colleague, ask.

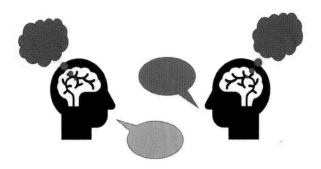

Figure 5.2 Make the Invisible Visible
In any conversation, there are typically multiple conversations going on. What's foreground is what we say. What's background is, for example, our inner dialogue, beliefs, unspoken assumptions, body-mindset, and worldview. When what your patient is saying is not congruent with body language, tone, tenor , and pitch, that's your cue to ask a generative question.

Tune In and Experience It Yourself

Take a moment and notice what is in the background of your awareness: the conversation you're having with yourself. You might notice, "I'm feeling some pressure to finish my charting so I can get enough sleep." Or, "I'm excited to practice some of this material tomorrow with my patients and thinking how to do it." Or, "My brain is tired. I'm overwhelmed." Bring it to the foreground by naming it.

What we can name, we can tame.

Don't wonder and make up your own answers or ignore your inner wisdom that is inspiring curiosity. For example:

I wonder...	Ask:
...what Mary means by the phrase _____?	Mary, what do you mean by the phrase _____?
...how they interpreted my statement?	What did you understand me to say?
...if Betty can process new information right now?	Betty, what's going on for you right now? What are you feeling? What are you thinking?
...what Paul's goals for treatment are?	Paul, what goals do you have regarding your treatment?
...what they have tried?	What have you tried?
...what they want?	What do you want? What is your highest hope?
...how this new treatment will fit into their life?	How might you fit this new healthcare plan into your day? How might you make sure to do this regimen every day?
...what actions they will take going forward?	What action are you going to take going forward? How can you take ownership for your health?
...what is getting in the way of following the treatment plan?	What do you think is making it difficult for you to follow the treatment plan? Or even better, What's helping you follow the treatment plan?

Trust your intuition. Consider the background questions you are asking yourself. If those questions are about someone else, resist the urge to answer them. Instead of drawing a conclusion based on your assumptions, ask the person. It will bring the information into the foreground for both of you and create shared understanding.

Generate New Knowledge

Asking questions that invite exploration outside our habitual ways of doing and understanding often results in new insights and new knowledge. This opens the door to new choices and potentially new behaviors. **What are you hoping to achieve today? What does ideal health look, feel, and sound like? What are you hoping I can do for you today? Imagine you are able to move and do all the activities you love, what does that look like? How have you accomplished "big things" in the past? What might we be missing? How might we make this happen? What gets in the way of taking your medication? When have you been successful at building a new habit?**

Inspire Possibilities

Generative questions can expand possibilities for people. For patients, they might inspire ideas to help them feel better, heal, or find a pathway through their crisis. For colleagues, they may lead to creative solutions, innovations, or break-through insights. If you find your patients or colleagues are resistant, stuck, or narrowly focused on the problem, ask generative questions that disrupt the way they are thinking and invite possibility. **What else might you try? What do others do in this situation? What do you want to happen here? What if…? How might you…? What outcome are you hoping for and what are all the possible ways of achieving that outcome? If three wishes could change everything for you, what would you wish for?**

If they're still stuck, back up and ask questions that make the invisible visible. Often what blocks our creative potential are invisible and unconscious influencers: assumptions, beliefs, rules, fears, and biases.

Applying Generative Questions in Healthcare

Generative questions empower patients to participate in their healing journey rather than be passive recipients of care. They inspire other healthcare professionals to stay open, connected, and creative. The following stories are examples of how generative questions can be powerful levers to support wellbeing, healing, and transitioning from cure to comfort. They are intended to catalyze your practice of asking generative questions.

Treatment Options

De'Ante arrives at the urgent care center. The Physician Assistant (PA), Juan asks, "What brings you here today?" De'Ante shows the PA this intensely itchy rash on his lower legs and describes his recent hike in the woods. De'Ante states, "I'm pretty sure this is poison ivy. I've just never had it this bad before." The PA finishes the history and physical, saying, "**What are you hoping for in this visit?**" De'Ante becomes animated, explaining, "Next weekend I'm going to be a groomsman in my fraternity brother's wedding—on the beach. We are all wearing linen shirts, shorts, and sandals. I need this rash to be gone by then!" Juan replies, "Got it! Let's blast this rash with topical and oral steroids, to get your legs ready for this wedding!" Juan now can align treatment options with De'Ante's goal.

Diagnostic Collaboration

Doctor Lin reviews a normal CT of abdomen and pelvis with the radiologist in the Emergency Department at a community hospital. Bridget is 21 years old and has right lower quadrant abdominal pain, nausea, and vomiting. Dr. Lin shares this normal finding with her. Bridget exclaims breathlessly, "It hurts so bad. I can't imagine walking out of here. It's got to be something. **How can we get more information?**" Considering the patient's condition and question, the EM doctor calls the surgeon, Dr. Khan, who is doing rounds in the hospital. He asks, **"What's the possibility this patient has appendicitis with a normal CT?"** Dr. Khan evaluates the patient who has physical signs of peritonitis and discusses treatment options, including surgery. Bridget agrees to an exploratory laparoscopy, where an inflamed appendix is discovered and removed.

Informed Consent

"It seems the first three rounds of chemotherapy have not been effective. The best option at this stage is to try a more aggressive chemotherapy. We would start with three treatments and give you medicine to manage the side effects," said Dr. Anison. **"What if that doesn't work?"** Jane asks. "Depending on your tolerance of the meds and your kidney function, we would try another round," the doctor responds. "What do you mean about my kidneys?" Jane asks, alarmed. "The more aggressive chemo would likely result in your kidneys shutting down. You might need dialysis, but that can be easily managed. We do it all the time," Dr. Anison responds. "I'd be on dialysis? No way!" exclaims Jane. "My brother had to go to the hospital every other day for months with dialysis. He had no life!" Dr. Anison pauses and shifts gears, "Let me back up Jane. **What is your understanding about the treatment recommendation I've shared with you?"**

Code Status Conversation

Matthew is admitted for pneumonia, again. The internal medicine hospitalist enters his room and sits down next to his bed. The hospitalist asks, **"May we talk for a few minutes? I want to** understand how you want your medical care to happen, now and in the future." Matthew agrees, and the hospitalist engages him in

51

a conversation using the following questions, "I see that you are a full code. **What does that mean to you?**" Following Matthew's response, the hospitalist says, "I'd like to talk with you about your wishes if you need life support. **What does life support mean to you? What are your wishes if your breathing or your heart were to stop, which are signs of natural death?**"

Terminal Illness and End of Life Issues

Dr. Jackson visits Betty in the hospital, "**How are you doing with all of this?**" Betty replies, "I hate coming to the hospital, but that's what I have to do when my breathing gets so bad." Dr. Jackson asks, "**If you weren't in the hospital, what would you be doing?**" After Betty's reply, Dr. Jackson asks, "**How would it feel to never have to come back to the hospital?**" "That would be amazing, but how can I do that?" After further dialogue, Dr. Jackson summarizes, "What I hear you saying, Betty, is that you don't want to return to the hospital for aggressive medical care. I hear you saying that you love your home, your gardens, and being home is what a good life looks like at this point in your life. **Did I get that right?**"

Betty agrees and Dr. Jackson continues, "I also have heard you say to me in past conversations that you know your lungs are 'pooping out,' and that you don't want to prolong the inevitable. So, I need to ask, **what does a good death look like through your eyes?**" Betty smiles, this was an easy question for her. "I want to be at home, with my family around me, with the drapes open, facing my beautiful backyard. I want it to feel like a party, or maybe, a gathering. I want them to be able to lean on each other when I die." Dr. Jackson replies, "What a beautiful image! When you are ready, I think the medical care that most aligns with that vision is hospice care. **What do you know about hospice?**"

Pre-Op

At 74, Jack is in excellent health. He and his wife, Lisa, take a long hike. That evening, Jack collapses with what Lisa suspects is a stroke. She rushes him to the hospital, and test results show 95% occlusion of the left carotid artery. Surgery is scheduled for the next day.

Lisa is at her husband's bedside when the surgeon walks in. "Morning, Jack," greets the doctor, and he nods to Lisa. **"How are you doing this morning?"** Jack has some muscle function back and is able to talk. The doctor follows, **"So, what do you think about doing surgery this morning?"** Looking puzzled, Jack replies, "You're the doctor. How should I know?" The doctor smiles, "I ask that question to help me understand how *you* are feeling about surgery. Whether you think it's a good idea, and where your emotions are." Jack replies, "Does it matter?" The doctor replies, "Actually, it does. Knowing what's going on for you helps me better assess and mitigate risks." Jack cracks a crooked smile, "I'm feeling scared and thankful that you know what you are doing. I trust you, Doc. I'm ready! Let's get this artery cleaned out."

Moving Past Deference or Implicit Authority

Jane has been Dr. Pandar's primary care patient for over 30 years. Diagnosed with advanced ovarian cancer eight months ago, she has been balancing chemotherapy with her weakened kidneys. She knows her cancer is terminal and wants to spend the time she has left with her family at home instead of coming in for additional treatments. Jane has already signed a DNR. She pleads, "Doctor, my oncologist doesn't get it. She's not listening to me."

Dr. Pandar calls her oncologist, Dr. Anison, who shares, "I think the more aggressive chemo could have some benefit. Jane should consider it. Kidney failure is common with this treatment, but dialysis is not a problem, we can manage it. I have had many patients in this situation before." **"How much additional time did those other patients gain with aggressive treatment?"** Dr. Pandar asks. "A few months, at best," replies Dr. Anison. "Were those other patients comfortable and at home most of that time?" asks Dr. Pandar. "They came in quite a bit due to side effects, but everyone is different," responds Dr. Anison. Dr. Pandar pauses, breathes, and asks, **"How does your treatment recommendation align with what matters most to Jane?"**

Family Issue

"Are you overriding my request?" Douglas demands authoritatively. His younger sister, Melanie, breathes deeply, twice, and replies, "I guess you can see it that way. I will not bring your clothes so you can leave the hospital today. Doug, you need to be here. I can see that you are confused. **What's going on for you right now?"** Doug bellows, "I don't even know. I can't keep it all straight in my head." Melanie replies, "I'd like to be with you. Please let me help support and advocate for you. **How can I help you review the information and keep it straight in your head?"**

Stressed Colleague

Chief of Staff and OB/GYN, Dr. Xavier Martinez, is worn out by a heavy schedule of meetings, made more challenging because they are virtual. At 7:00 am, he is reviewing hospital performance metrics with the health system COO and Quality Director. The COO reflects, "Dr. Martinez, what's up with the C-Section rates? They are really shooting up!" Dr. Martinez fires back sarcastically, "I dunno Christine. We have 42 OB/GYNs on staff, have you asked any of them?" His heart is pounding;

he folds his arms, clamps his mouth shut, and considers turning off the camera on his laptop. Towards the end of the meeting, he remembers the practice of tuning in.

He pauses and takes a deep breath; Dr. Martinez gets curious. **"Where am I?"** he asks himself. He notices his tight muscles and abdomen, his clenched jaw and furrowed brow. With slow, deliberate breathing, he softens his body. He asks, **"What's going on for me right now? What about that question triggered me?"** His administrative role limits his obstetric practice, and he doesn't feel connected to the other OBs in the hospital. He acknowledges that a blend of personal and specialty-based pride contributed to his brusque response. Then he thinks, **"What do I know about our cesarian section rates? What questions might I ask the 42 OB/GYNs on staff to better understand this issue? What other data may exist for my review?"**

After the meeting and day of patient care, he stops by Christine's office. "Christine, sorry about my response in that meeting. **Can I have a do-over?"** He asks with a sheepish grin. "Of course!" Christine replies. "I'm sorry I put you on the spot. But it did get me thinking about what questions we might ask the OB/GYNs on staff. Let's talk!"

Generative Questions, The First of Two Practices

Asking generative questions helps us uncover new information and builds rapport. Generative questions make the invisible visible, move background to foreground, and help us see our patients more completely. In the next chapter, we will explore positive framing, the second practice for turning our conversations into ones worth having.

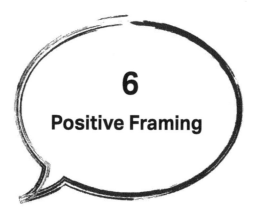

6
Positive Framing

"The optimist sees the donut; the pessimist sees the hole."
—*Oscar Wilde*

The story that follows is in the voice of one of the authors who lived it, Jackie Stavros:

On the eve of Paul's 45th birthday, after eight critical days in the hospital, we await his biopsy results. Dr. Ferahi greets us with her tight firm smile. She is focused and direct, "Paul has Stage 4 Lymphoma." All I hear is Stage 4. My mind goes blank, panic takes over, and I am having trouble breathing while trying desperately to hold back tears. This has to be wrong. My husband is young, fit, and strong. We had a three-week hiking vacation planned and two young children at home. We have lots of plans for the future. Losing him right now is inconceivable. The doctor continues talking about the results, treatments, and tests, but I've stopped hearing what she is saying after the words, "Stage 4." My thoughts are a jumble. I looked at Paul. His eyes are wide, and his face is white as a ghost. I'm scared, but he is clearly terrified. That's when I remember that this isn't all about me. Whatever I am feeling, I knew that in that moment that he was feeling it 100 times over.

Dr. Ferahi keeps repeating that Stage 4 with this type of cancer has a 50% survival rate. I finally hear her and ask, "So Stage 4 is not terminal?" She repeats, "He has a 50% chance of surviving. And, we have a chemo cocktail and regimen that I believe Paul can get through. I ask again, "This Stage 4, there is a cure, and he can survive?" She kindly and patiently repeats, "We have a plan that we believe will provide Paul with the best possible outcome. I would like to explain this chemo regimen and give you some time to take it all in."

She explains the details of how this 24-week chemo regimen will work. Then, she asks if there are any immediate questions. Paul still has said nothing. My mind is racing with questions but where to start. She asks us both to just *pause* for a moment, take a *deep breath*, and sit with everything. She will come back in a short while to check in on us and see what other questions we have.

She leaves the hospital room, and I rush to sit on the bed with Paul and just hold him. The room is eerily quiet. My mind feels like it is blindly racing through thick fog. I want to ask Paul how he is feeling, but I know that is a stupid question. The answer is all too obvious—he is scared, nervous, and angry all blended into one. I know that if I get him talking about the diagnosis, the conversation will quickly spiral down into a pit of despair and anguish. In a moment of desperation, I latch on to one subject that I know might get Paul in a positive focus.

"We have to tell the kids, Paul. **How can we be honest with them and also help them find some understanding and meaning out of whatever happens with this?**" I ask. My question catches him off guard. I watch Paul's face carefully as my question sinks in. Very slowly his face shifts from a look of hopelessness to one of thoughtful consideration. Paul loves our children more than anything, and he takes his job as a dad and role model very seriously. Finally, he says quietly, "You're right, we need to be careful how we handle this. Whether we like it or not, they need to learn how to deal with adversity. And, we can't promise them that I am not going to die."

For the rest of the evening, we talk about how we are going to break the news to the kids. Since he will not be going home from the hospital with me, I am going to inform the kids. Paul's demeanor shifts from helpless patient to concerned father who is going to need his family in the fight of his life. His perspective becomes determined. Instead of focusing on his cancer, we decide to engage the kids in creating a healing environment at home and working together to support his treatment, envisioning it being successful.

While this news is devastating, Paul recalls his mother's words, "It is a parent's responsibility to help their children become adults. And an important part of that is the ability to handle suffering with grace." By the time I get home, not only do I have a frame for my conversation with the kids, but I feel ready for this difficult conversation that will be one worth having. I want to support my kids, move from fear to courage, despair to hope, hopelessness to action, and illness to wellbeing. We immediately begin creating the best living environment to support his treatment journey and survival.

Positive Framing

What Paul and Jackie did was create a positive frame for conversations with their children. In the introduction, you learned that positive framing is talking about desired outcomes instead of focusing on problems. It is also about shifting your thinking toward possibilities and highest hopes. Such framing provides a structure for aligning generative questions, behavior, and actions that will support that envisioned outcome. This simple shift in focus typically gives us access to the energy needed to support action.

In the introduction, we shared the flipping technique (see Figure 1.3). For Paul and Jackie, the steps look like this:

- **Name It:** Paul has Stage 4 cancer.
- **Flip It:** Paul does not have Stage 4 cancer; he's in remission.
- **Frame It:** We are living fully today; all of us contributing to a positive environment and anticipating Paul will be in the surviving 50%.

Notice that the frame is not simply putting on rose-colored glasses and imagining everything will be fine. It's a frame that supports being fully alive right now, fueling positivity and meaning, creating conditions for the best possible outcome to happen, and hoping for the best. A positive frame gives people a sense of possibility and empowers them to take positive action to support desired outcomes. That can be powerfully healing in and of itself. Such a perspective gives a person the best fighting chance when they are dealing with illness. It boosts their immune system and allows them to stay in a connect body-mindset.

Generative questions are often used in the process of creating a positive frame and then again to help people discover a path towards that desired outcome. Jackie asked Paul a generative question that resulted in a frame for her conversation with the kids.[37] Additional generative questions related to the frame helped them create an ultra-clean home to reduce risk of infection and a positive atmosphere filled with activities that inspired love and wellbeing for the entire family.

Applying Positive Framing in Healthcare

As a healthcare professional, you can use generative questions to encourage patients or colleagues to flip their focus from problem to desired outcome. Your questions can allow individuals to get clear on what they really want and what is important to them. It helps patients realize the locus of control lies within themselves, which is the foundation of self-efficacy.

The following stories illustrate how you can work with your patients and colleagues to create a positive frame around healthcare situations. Through each story, you'll see how to flip a problem and arrive at a frame for a conversation worth having.

Goals of Care and Code Status

Betty hoped her cough and fatigue would lessen, but over the past two days her breathing has worsened. Betty won't call 911, she knows driving isn't a good idea, so she calls her neighbor Lucy.

Lucy kindly takes Betty into the Emergency Department (ED). Betty keeps suggesting that Lucy leave, but Lucy offers to be a second set of eyes and ears during the visit. Betty nods and breathes laboriously, as if sucking through a narrow straw. Nurse, lab tech, EKG tech, radiology tech with portable x-ray machine, the intern, then resident, and then attending physician of the ED stream through her exam room.

A young man in a white coat enters the room, and briskly states, "Ms. Manolo, we are going to keep you here for a few days. I have called the hospitalists to come see you, and they will get you tucked in upstairs. In the meantime, we will continue treating your COPD, so hopefully you will start feeling better soon.

"I just have a few final questions. If your breathing were to get worse, would you want to have a breathing tube placed and be put on a ventilator?" Betty says, "Um, yes. I was feeling fine a few days ago!"

"If your heart were to stop, do you want all the interventions to bring you back to life?" He asks. "I guess so," Betty muses. He continues, "Even if that means CPR, which may break your ribs, and you might need intensive care services?" She replies, "Well…yes, if I can come back."

He presses on, "Do you have a DPOA—a legal document, a paper that states who will speak for you if you cannot speak for yourself for medical decision making?" Betty stammers, "I don't know. I've never been asked that." Betty looks at Lucy, and the resident turns to Lucy, "Are you her medical DPOA?" Lucy looks decidedly uncomfortable and shakes her head no.

Betty sits bewildered, trying to reconcile the young man's initial statement of being in the hospital for a few days, with these subsequent questions suggesting dying may be imminent.

Before she can ask a clarifying question, he states, "So you want to be a full code. I'll send the social worker in with DPOA paperwork. You should really get that done and on file, I mean, your COPD is not going to get better!" and leaves the room.

A heavy silence falls between Lucy and Betty. Betty looks up, tears in her eyes and asks, "Am I that bad? Is my heart going to stop?" Lucy reassures Betty that she will get better, and the doctor is just completing required paperwork.

Before Betty's nervous system was hijacked in the code status conversation, she was beginning to feel better with the oxygen. Had the young man understood the power of framing a conversation, he might have had a different conversation. Here's how he might have flipped the focus of the interaction:

- **Name It**: COPD is exacerbated.
- **Flip It**: She breathes freely.
- **Frame It**: Hospitalization is short and provides effective treatment.

You can see how the questions that arise from this frame are more life-enhancing. For example: **"What does living well mean for you? How can we best support that here in the hospital? What information do you need to understand Code Status?"**

Patient Barriers to Taking Medications

Joe's diabetic labs once again show that his blood sugars are dangerously high; Dr. Miranda Varga, his family doctor, suspects he's still not taking his medications. For the last year, she has focused on trying to get him to appreciate the organ damage persistently high blood sugars can cause. Telling him about eventual blindness, kidney failure, heart attacks, strokes, life-threatening infections, and amputations has not been a motivator. Joe always looks ashamed, but he gives Dr. Varga the same excuse: he doesn't like taking the meds because he ends up in the bathroom with diarrhea. As a 32-year-old elementary teacher, diarrhea does NOT fit into his schedule! Dr. Varga decides to flip the conversation.

- **Name It:** Joe is not taking his medicine and has uncontrolled diabetes.
- **Flip It:** Joe's diabetes is well controlled.
- **Frame It:** Joe is able to avoid significant organ damage and do the things he loves for the rest of his life because he's able to keep his diabetes controlled.

For most patients with diabetes, healthcare professionals connect the untreated disease to its long-term debilitating outcomes. This negative, deficit-based focus is scary for patients, putting them below the line, and projects too far into the future for patients to feel motivated to adhere to today's treatment plan. With a new frame, Dr. Varga asks generative questions to start a different conversation: **"What else keeps you from taking your meds? How might your diet be related to your diarrhea? What other medicines can we try? With the proposed medicine changes, who can be your accountability partner? What do you value about your health? What are your favorite activities to do? What activities do you want to continue doing in the next five years? Imagine you are at the end of your life, and you are looking back upon it, what are you grateful that your body was able to do for you?"** In asking these questions, and deeply listening to Joe's answers, Dr. Varga can easily link the need for diabetes treatment to the patient's motivations and desires.

Treatment Approach

Rich messed up his knee playing hockey and could hardly walk. At the surgeon's office, Rich explains how the injury occurred, describes the pain, and what he can no longer do, while the surgeon examines him. Rich keeps complaining and talking about loss, until the surgeon interrupts him and asks, **"What is it you want to be able to do down the road? What's on your bucket list? How does your knee need to function for you in the future?"** Rich thought about it. "I love to hike and travel. I want to explore and climb Machu Picchu." The surgeon smiles, and says, "Let's work on a healing process to support your knee and allow you to do those things." Rich shifts from fixating on the injury to focusing on the healing plan.

- **Name It:** Rich's knee hurts and isn't working.
- **Flip It:** Rich's knee works and doesn't hurt.
- **Frame It:** Rich can travel and climb amazing wonders of the world.

Addressing Healthcare Risks

Constance, a nurse practitioner (NP) is talking to Hans, an 86-year-old man, who recently fell. He has essential tremor, restless legs syndrome, reflux, and an enlarged prostate. He got dizzy, lost his balance, and fell while peering through his binoculars on a recent bird walk. Constance responds, "Well, at your age you shouldn't be craning your neck like that. I'm afraid your next fall could really hurt you. I recommend you stop birding." He responds, "But I love to birdwatch. I take guided walks in regional parks almost every weekend. Spotting a bird high in a rustling tree is what I live for!" If the conversation ends here, Hans is likely to ignore the NP's advice and fall again or follow the advice and lose a great joy in his life. Here's a way for the NP to create a positive frame:

- **Name It:** Hans cannot birdwatch safely.
- **Flip It:** Hans may birdwatch safely.
- **Frame It:** Following specific precautions, Hans can continue to do what he loves—birdwatching.

Again, generative questions arise almost naturally with this frame. **"What strategies could help you look high into the trees safely? Do you have bird watching friends with you? How might you engage some of these people in supporting you on these walks? Is there a friend or family member willing to accompany you, serving as an extra set of eyes and physical support as you walk over uneven terrain?"**

Turning Significant Loss into Possibility

Rod, a shift nurse, is trying to uplift a patient after an accident destroyed her eyesight. The patient says, "I don't want to live without seeing! I wish I'd died in the accident." Instead of trying to convince her otherwise, he reframes the conversation.

- **Name It:** Patient doesn't want to live without her eyesight.

- **Flip It:** Patient does want to live, even without her eyesight.

- **Frame It:** Life is meaningful, and she has a way to contribute positively.

Rod begins, "I can only imagine how devastating it is to lose your eyesight and how life might seem meaningless without it. **What kinds of things have been most meaningful for you in your life?**" The conversation initially centers on things she could see before, but Rod gently asks, "**What else?**" The patient moves beyond emphasizing vision and into relationships with her family, contributions she was making with her volunteer work with the homeless, and her deep joy of music and dance. By the time the conversation is over, the patient has relived many life experiences of joy and meaning, which were not dependent on her sight. For the first time since the accident, she feels hope.

Irascible Patient

The nurses, housekeeping, and interns are complaining about the patient in room 302. He is critical of everything and everyone, continuously complains, and constantly demands attention. Everyone is beginning to ignore the buzzer for 302, which makes the patient even more irritable. The Unit Manager calls a huddle to discuss this with staff.

- **Name It:** No one wants to deal with the patient in 302.

- **Flip It:** Everyone is willing to deal with the patient in 302.

- **Frame It:** Staff have a way to understand and respond to the patient in 302 that is meaningful and life-giving.

The manager begins by acknowledging that the patient in 302, Mr. Bee, is difficult, and the staff reaction is understandable. She goes on, "At the same time, we hold ourselves to a level of excellence in service and care that requires us to serve even the most difficult patients. **What do we know about him and his support system? What might explain his need for constant attention, and his behaviors that push everyone away? What else might explain it? What can we do as a team to understand and respond to this patient in meaningful and life-giving ways? What questions might we ask him to gain some understanding?"**

Positive Framing as a Wellbeing Factor

You will find it effective and affirming to use positive framing in your conversations. Research in positive psychology provides evidence concerning the benefits of a healthy positivity ratio.[38] People enter healthcare professions to make a difference in the lives of others, relieve suffering, and facilitate health and wellbeing. With positive framing, healthcare professionals can support desired outcomes, articulating and aligning medical care with the patient's goals to live their best life now. It can also raise the positivity ratio in healthcare interactions.

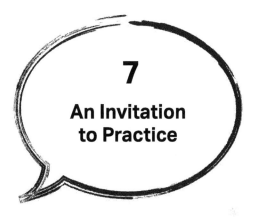

7
An Invitation
to Practice

"Knowledge is of no value unless you put it into practice."
—*Anton Chekhov*

David Cooperrider said, "We live in worlds our conversations create." Each conversation we have has the potential for connection, understanding, appreciation, and healing. This is true of our internal dialogue as well as our external conversations with patients, families, and colleagues. The more adept we become at conversations worth having, the more effective we will be at manifesting this potential and improving the lives of our patients, their families, and our lives as well.

Throughout this book, we've offered ways healthcare professionals and caregivers can engage patients in creating images, actions, and decisions that align with the patient's concept of health and wellbeing. We've offered the practices of tuning in, asking generative questions, and creating a positive frame to support conversations worth having. Using these skills in conversations will allow you to better understand the needs of your patients and support their healing, from the diabetic man's medications to Paul and his family finding their way forward through the challenges of Stage 4 lymphoma treatment.

What might it mean for your patients, their family members, and your colleagues to pause…breathe…get curious, and follow that curiosity toward a desired outcome? For the patient, **how might their ability to ask generative questions empower them to fully understand and participate in their healthcare?** For the caregiver, **how might envisioning the future with their loved one help them through challenging moments?** For the healthcare professional, **how might these practices impact the effectiveness of your work and satisfaction with daily interactions? How might it influence your personal life, family, friends, and communities?**

The summary and exercise that follows invites you to breathe life into that potential. The list of generative questions in the Appendix and the flipping worksheet at the end of this chapter are resources to enhance your capacity to use these practices. Additional resources are available at http://www. conversationsworthhaving.today, where you can deepen your understanding through webinars and customized workshops, which include certification as a *Conversations Worth Having* coach, trainer, and practitioner.

A Snapshot for Fostering Conversations Worth Having

The concepts in this book can be easily summarized:

- **Harness the power of conversations.** There are four types of conversations, and each one influences our state and the outcomes of the interaction. Conversations above the line invite wellbeing, connection, creativity, expansion, and possibility. Conversations below the line generate and reinforce states of protection, hopelessness, defensiveness, disease, and disempowerment. For healthy relationships, strive for a positive (above the line) to negative (below the line) interactions ratio of 4:1. Given the negativity bias of the human brain, achieving this ratio takes deliberate effort and practice.[39]

- **Be intentional: tune in.** As healthcare professionals, our body-mindset influences our reactions and responses to the people around us: patients, family members, team members, and colleagues. When we are above the line, we initiate conversations worth having with greater ease. Tuning in by pausing, breathing, and getting curious primes us to be deliberate in our conversations and to use the two simple practices.

- **Ask generative questions.** The questions we ask effect change the moment we ask them. Asking such questions runs counter to the way many of us have been trained. They are open-ended, seek depth over brevity, and embrace "what is" without a covert agenda. They widen the frame, often giving a broader context for diagnosis and treatment. Generative questions make the invisible visible, create shared understanding, generate new knowledge, and inspire possibilities.

- **Create a positive frame.** You can shift problem-focused challenges into opportunities for quality care, quality living, and positive patient outcomes. Positive framing allows us to intentionally focus on desired outcomes and the patient's possible future. Use Flipping—name it, flip it, frame it—to help you explore problems and issues and reframe them into desired outcomes.

To summarize these concepts in action, let's check in on Betty and Dr. Jackson one last time. Two years after her original diagnosis, Betty meets with Dr. Jackson, bringing peonies from her garden. Betty beams with pride—loving her garden's bounty. Dr. Jackson thanks Betty, and says, "With such beautiful flowers as a result, no wonder you love your garden so much! How is it going?" Betty shares that she needs to rest more frequently between tasks. Dr. Jackson states, "Betty, that is what I suspected. Your oxygen level is dropping. Today at rest, your oxygen saturation was 90%. Two years ago, your resting oxygen level was 95%. When I had Conner walk you around a bit, it dropped to 84% in less than one minute. I believe it is a lack of oxygen that is making you tired and needing to rest more. I think you need supplemental oxygen to breathe and function well."

Betty is taken aback. Her face must have betrayed her thoughts. Dr. Jackson asks, "**Hey, what's going on in your head right now? What does wearing oxygen mean to you?**" Betty pauses, and then reminds herself that Dr. Jackson really cares. So, she says, "I don't want to look different, like a doddering old lady! I'm afraid of how clunky it will be, and how I can manage at home. How can I drag a big oxygen tank around in my backyard?"

Dr. Jackson takes in all of Betty's statements and says, "I really admire how you share your thoughts and feelings with me. Knowing what matters most to you helps me to figure out the best way to care for you. I hear you saying that you want to continue to work in your garden and be as independent and functional as possible. **Did I hear that right?**" Betty nods and Dr. Jackson continues, "I believe that extra oxygen, if packaged in a way that is portable, will allow you to continue doing the activities you love." She gestures to the flowers on the counter, "I definitely want you to keep growing these beautiful peonies!"

Betty laughs, and replies, "Doc, I know that my lungs are just getting weaker, even though I'm not around smoke anymore. I've been thinking about the questions you asked me before, and glad that I haven't had to return to the hospital. I am done with that. I want to live in my home and enjoy the rest of my life in the beauty I've created. That feels right. I have looked at the hospice information you gave me, and as long as I can still have you as my doctor, then I am ready to ask for the help of hospice. I remember you saying that needing help isn't a weakness, but a reality of being human. I'm ready." Dr. Jackson reaches out and squeezes Betty's hand, saying, "I'll be with you the whole way."

Your Turn to Try It

Take a few moments to consider a challenging patient situation or a conversation with another healthcare professional. As you think about the situation:

- **Tune in:** Take a moment to pause and check in. When you think about the other person in the conversation, do you shift above the line (toward connect) or below the line (toward protect)? Take a deep breath. Feel your lungs and belly expand as you fill up with fresh air. Soften and release as you exhale. Notice what shifts or changes as you breathe. Bring some gentle curiosity to your state and situation: What are you feeling/noticing in your body? What don't you know about how your patient might be feeling/noticing? How about your colleague? Now, get curious about the other person: What background information might you be missing? What assumptions are you making? What story are you telling yourself about the other? What other stories might explain the situation? Keep breathing.

- **Ask generative questions:** What don't you know for certain? What are you curious about? What questions might you ask? For example, "What's a normal day look like for you? What relationships give you the greatest joy? What energizes you? What are your goals?" Such questions allow you to expand your understanding of another's world. What information will broaden your view so that you can be of greatest service to the other person. What questions will make the invisible visible? Create shared understanding? Generate new knowledge? Inspire possibilities?

- **Use a positive frame:** How might you apply flipping to create a positive frame for the conversation? If you are clear on the other person's goals, what are a few possible frames you could use in your next conversation with them? If you're not sure of their goals, how might you engage them in flipping their focus and clarifying the outcomes they are seeking? Validate what you have heard by reflecting back to ensure shared understanding of the patient's desired outcomes.

In addition to interactions healthcare professionals have with patients and their caregivers, think of all the other conversations you have with colleagues and families, in your office, in the breakroom, the hallways, and in meetings. Imagine if each of these conversations was one worth having. How might generative questions and positive framing influence your quality improvement meetings, medical staff meetings, Board of Director sessions, staff meetings and others? How might increasing your daily dose of conversations worth having influence your positive to negative interaction ratio? How would this influence your energy and resilience? How might conversations worth having sustain you and your capacity to practice medicine?

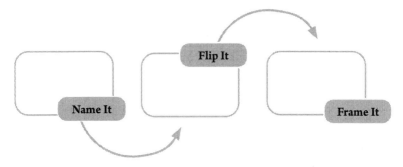

Our Call to Action

As a healthcare professional, you are engaged in conversations (with yourself and others) all day long. Conversations worth having are essential to delivering quality healthcare. Deliberately applying these two simple practices amplifies your awareness of what is good, possible, and meaningful in your work and relationships. May your conversations create a world of wellbeing, hope, and possibility for patients, for colleagues, and for yourself.

Appendix:
Sample Questions

Make the Invisible Visible

Questions to ask yourself:

- Where am I? (Above the Line/Below the Line)
- What's going on for me right now (body, mind, emotions)?
- What about that question triggered me?
- What don't I know? What might I be missing?
- What assumptions am I making?
- What role is my ego playing in this situation?
- How might hidden biases be influencing my action(s)?
- …and what else?
- What am I observing that is out of sync: an expression, a tone, a statement, or an intuition?
- What unspoken assumptions, beliefs, or cultural norms may be influencing their actions?

Questions to ask others:

- What do you value in this situation? What's your perspective?
- What motivates you?
- What outcome are you hoping for?
- What specific concerns do you have?
- What's going on for you right now?
- What are you thinking/feeling?

- What led you to that conclusion?
- What informed your decision?
- What does your support system look like?
- What does living well mean for you?
- What is your highest hope?
- What kinds of things have been most meaningful for you in your life?
- What does a good death look like through your eyes?

Create Shared Understanding

- In our discussion, we've agreed to cover _____ today. How does that sound to you?
- What is your understanding of your health condition and the tests we've run?
- What activities are important for you to continue doing?
- What matters most to you at this point in your care?
- What does quality of life mean for you?
- What are your priorities?
- What does a "good life" look like to you?
- What do you mean by the phrase _____?
- I heard you say _____. What did I miss? What did I misunderstand?
- What else would you like me to know that I haven't asked?
- What is your understanding of the information I've shared?
- What will help you follow the treatment plan?

- What might get in the way?
- What action are you going to take going forward?

Generate New Knowledge

Questions to ask yourself:

- What might I ask colleagues to better understand this issue?
- How might we make this happen?
- What other data and information exists to inform us?

Questions to ask others:

- What are you hoping to accomplish in our time together?
- Who might accompany you to be an extra set of eyes and ears?
- What does ideal health look, feel, and sound like to you?
- What is it you want to be able to do down the road?
- What's made you successful in following the treatment plan?
- How might you fit this new healthcare plan into your day?
- How do you motivate yourself?
- How have you approached challenges in the past?
- When have you been successful at building a new habit?

Inspire Possibilities

- When our work together goes well, what conditions make it possible?
- What do you want to happen here?
- What are possible ways of achieving your desired outcome?
- What else could we try?
- What do others do in this situation?
- With the proposed changes to your treatment plan, who might be your accountability partner?
- If three wishes changed everything for you, what would your wishes be?
- How can you best share your condition with others that respect your boundaries and support you in living well?
- What other modalities might we consider for your treatment?
- What can we do as a team to understand and respond to this patient in meaningful and life-affirming ways?

Generative questions, by definition, are open-ended. The following words will help you ask questions with a generative spirit:

- What if…?
- How might you…?
- How might I…?
- Where can I…?
- What examples…?

Notes

Chapter 1

1. M. Bremer, "The Paradox of Leading Change," OCAI.org. Available 11/23/2021 at https://www.ocai-online.com/blog/positive-change-with-appreciative-questions, accessed on 01/30/2022.
2. E. J. Pace, N. J. Somerville, C. Enyioha, J. P. Allen, L. C. Lemon, and C. W. Allen, "Effects of a Brief Psychosocial Intervention on Inpatient Satisfaction: A Randomized Controlled Trial," *Family Medicine*, 2017 Oct;49(9):675–678.
3. N. Singh Ospina, K. A. Phillips, R. Rodriguez-Gutierrez, A. Castaneda-Guarderas, M. R. Gionfriddo, M. E. Branda, and V. M. Montori, "Eliciting the Patient's Agenda—Secondary Analysis of Recorded Clinical Encounters," *Journal of General Internal Medicine*, 2019 Jan;34(1):36–40. doi: 10.1007/s11606-018-4540-5. Epub 2018 Jul 2.
4. N. Singh Ospina, K. A. Phillips, et al.
5. Sara Berg, "Empathy: A Critical Ally in Battling Physician Burnout," AMA.org. Available 12/29/20 at https://www.ama-assn.org/practice-management/physician-health/empathy-critical-ally-battling-physician-burnout.
6. P. Ranjan, A. Kumari, and A. Chakrawarty, "How Can Doctors Improve their Communication Skills?," *Journal of Clinical and Diagnostic Research*, 2015;9(3):JE01-JE4. Available 12/29/20 at https://greatergood.berkeley.edu/article/item/building_empathy_in_healthcare.
7. Jackie Stavros and Cheri Torres, *Conversations Worth Having: Using Appreciative Inquiry to Fuel Productive and Meaningful Engagement*, Second Edition (Oakland, CA: Berrett-Koehler Publishing, 2022).
8. Stavros and Torres, page 31.
9. These two practices are based on Appreciative Inquiry (AI), which is one of the most effectively used approaches for fostering positive change and dramatically improving the outcomes of your conversation. To learn more about these AI practices and its 5 core principles, see *Conversations Worth Having: Using Appreciative Inquiry to Fuel Productive and Meaningful Engagement*, Second Edition.
10. Empirical studies confirm that this produces a positive climate and significantly higher performance. Kim Cameron, Positive Leadership (San Francisco: Berrett-Koehler, 2012), and the Center for Positive Organizations; see http://positiveorgs.bus.umich.edu. Also, Michele McQuaid, *The Change Lab 2019 Workplace Survey*.
11. Francesca Gino, "The Business Case for Curiosity," *Harvard Business Review*, September-October 2018.
12. Stavros and Torres, pages 80–89.

13. Stavros and Torres, page 84.
14. To learn more about Appreciative Inquiry, visit AI Commons: https://appreciativeinquiry.champlain.edu/. The "AI Commons" is a place for everyone with an interest in Appreciative Inquiry (AI) and positive change.
15. You will find the more in-depth research and explanation of the AI Principles in Stavros and Torres, *Conversations Worth Having*.
16. To learn more about the AI Principles, see Chapter 5: What's Driving Your Conversation in Stavros and Torres, *Conversations Worth Having*.
17. Martin Seligman is a pioneer in the positive psychology field, and the theory of wellbeing and human flourishing. To learn more about how this field developed, visit www.pursuit-of-happiness.org/history-of-happiness/martin-seligman-psychology/. Also, David Rock, *Your Brain at Work* (NYC: Harper Business, 2020).
18. Barbara Fredrickson, "What Good Are Positive Emotions?," *Rev. General Psychology* 2, no. 30, September 1998, 300–319, and Barbara Fredrickson, "The Role of Positive Emotions in Positive Psychology: The Broaden-and-Build Theory of Positive Emotions," *American Psychologist* 56, no. 3, 2001, 218–26.
19. Barbara Fredrickson's research indicates that we need a minimum of a 3:1 ratio of positive emotions to negative emotions in order to stay healthy and vital. Fredrickson, *Positivity*. Marcial Losada and Emily Heaphy's research shows that high-performing teams actually have a 6:1 ratio: "The Role of Positivity and Connectivity in the Performance of Business Teams: A Nonlinear Dynamics Model," *American Behavioral Scientist* 47, no. 6, February 2004, 740–65.

Chapter 2
20   Stavros and Torres, Figure 2.2, page 33.

Chapter 3
21   D. M. Zulman, M. C. Haverfield, J. G. Shaw, et al., "Practices to Foster Physician Presence and Connection With Patients in the Clinical Encounter," *JAMA*, 2020;323(1):70–81.
22   D. Safran, D. Taira, W. Rogers, M. Kosinski, J. Ware, and A. Tarlov, "Linking primary care performance to outcomes of care.," *Journal of Family Practice*, 1995;47(3):213–220.
23   P. Ranjan, A. Kumari, and A. Chakrawart, "How Can Doctors Improve their Communication Skills?," *Journal of Clinical and Diagnostic Research*, 2015;9(3):JE01-JE4.
24   Stavros and Torres, page 136. See also, University of California, Los Angeles, "New UCLA Imagine Study First to Show Placebo Alters Brain Function in Individuals with Major Depression," *Science Daily*, January 2, 2002, https://www.sciencedaily.com/releases/2002/01/020102074543.htm.

25 BJ Fogg, TEDx: Forget Big Change, Start with a Tiny Habit. Available 1/21/21 at https://www.youtube.com/watch?v=AdKUJxjn-R8.

Chapter 4

26 Ego definition from Oxford Dictionary accessed on 04/13/2022 at https://www.oxfordreference.com/.
27 N. Singh Ospina, K. A. Phillips, et al.
28 Amy Windover, Adrienne Boissy, Thomas Rice, Timothy Gilligan, Vincente Velez and James Merlino, "The REDE model of healthcare communication: Optimizing relationship as a therapeutic agent," *Journal of Patient Experience*, Vol 1, Issue 1, 2014, pages 8–13.
29 Carol Dweck, *Mindset: The New Psychology of Success* (NY: Ballantine, 2016).
30 Daniel Kahneman, *Thinking Fast and Slow* (NY: Farrar, Straus, and Giroux, 2011), pages 21–30. A wonderful and practical application of Kahneman's work is explored by Matthew E. May, *Winning the Brain Game: Fixing the 7 Fatal Flaws of Thinking* (NY: McGraw-Hill, 2016).
31 Our emotional landscape, our physical state, and our mindset.
32 HeartMath research demonstrates that this is a powerful first step in being able to shift from a downward spiral to an upward neurological positive feedback loop—from incoherence to coherence. Find all research by the HeartMath Institute at https://www.heartmath.org/research/research-library/.
33 Andrew Huberman, neuroscientist and head of Madefor Advisory Board, Madefor's member communication, January 20. 2021, https://www.getmadefor.com.
34 Fredrickson, "What good are positive emotions?"

Chapter 5

35 Stavros and Torres, pages 136–138.
36 Stavros and Torres, page 72.

Chapter 6

37 See the full story and generative questions asked in Chapter 8: Any Time, Any Place, Any Situation in Stavros and Torres, pages 160–164.
38 Stavros and Torres, pages 143–147.

Chapter 7

39 See further details about the neuroscience behind this work in Stavros and Torres, Chapter 7.

CWH Offerings

Though the practices are simple, we know shifting our habits of conversation is not easy. To support you, those of us working to create a worldwide movement to generate positive change, one conversation at a time, are developing products to support you.

Conversation Bootcamps

We offer basic training and specialized trainings. Our Conversation Bootcamp focuses on deepening your appreciation for and experience of tuning in and using the two practices. Strategic Conversations uses the practices to support strategic planning, alignment, and goal achievement. We also offer a range of bootcamps that focus the training for specific industries or sectors, such as healthcare, wellbeing, and education.

CWH Certification

For those interested in joining the growing community of practitioners who can teach and facilitate conversations worth having and strategic conversations, we offer certification.

Self-directed, On-Demand Training

Learn and practice at your own pace with our self-directed On-Demand Conversation Bootcamps.

Monday Kickstarters

Practice flipping problems into positive frames and asking generative questions. These live 30-minute 6-week sessions occur throughout the year. Sessions are recorded and available on our Vimeo channel. You can also read the outcomes on our blog.

Supporting Products and Resources

Download our conversation toolkits. Play the *CWH Shift This!* card game with your colleagues to make learning to ask questions fun and easy. Use our other games, posters, and journals to make practice and development of new habits sticky! Check our webiste routinely for new offerings.

Learn more at cwh.today

About the Authors

Elizabeth Warner, MD FACP CPE is an internal medicine physician, improvement system coach, healthcare leader and president of Warner Well Being—committed to the flourishing of humans in healthcare. Dr. Warner received her MD from Michigan State University College of Human Medicine with Alpha Omega Alpha distinction. Her clinical experience spans primary care, hospital and nursing home medicine, geriatric care and palliative medicine. Her passion for learning and leading has guided her to training in improvement systems, positive psychology and organizational development, motivational interviewing and relationship-centered communication. She applies all of her knowledge to serve patients, healthcare leaders and organizations to transform into sustainable systems. Her public speaking experience ranges from custom multi-day training sessions to inspirational keynote addresses spanning transformational healthcare, improvement systems, humanism in medicine and resilience in healthcare. She believes that sustainable change in healthcare requires different behaviors, habits, processes and systems, grounded in principles of courageous leadership. These actions must happen internally, interpersonally, and at every level of organizations. Dr. Warner has hope in the potential of humans to co-create a thriving world of healthcare. warnerwellbeing@gmail.com.

Fasiha Haq is a veteran in the healthcare and life sciences sector and has spent over three decades working directly with patients, physicians, administrators, and global corporate organizations to bridge the science of clinical practice with the art of clinical care. She has provided training and mentoring to many healthcare professionals, at every stage of their career, on the intrapersonal and interpersonal skills critical for forging meaningful connections, building trust, and resolving conflicts in high stakes, time constrained environments. Her recent focus has been on application- based learning that helps residents and interns navigate the challenging hierarchy of healthcare teams. Complimenting her scientific and business expertise with certifications in Emotional Intelligence, Behavioral Psychology, Appreciative Inquiry, and Positive Psychology, she partners with forward thinking organizations to chart a course through institutional complexities and deliver high impact solutions. This has included convening diverse stakeholders such as policy makers, administrators, physicians and patients to collectively design realistic roadmaps that elevate the quality of care and improve both physician and patient satisfaction.

Known for her creative and playful spirit she thrives on making learning simple, fun, and highly practical, integrating experiential learning and application into even the most dense material. fasiha@conversationsworthhaving.today

Cheri Torres, Ph.D. As CEO of Collaborative by Design, Cheri partners with people to catalyze positive change in workplaces and communities. The two simple practices she introduces give leaders and teams the power to strengthen relationships, expand possibilities, and increase productivity and engagement through everyday conversation. These practices are grounded in neuroscience, positive psychology, and Appreciative Inquiry, one of the most widely used approaches for systems change. She's worked with thousands of leaders and teams around the world to support high performance, engagement, culture transformation, and organizational success.

As an author and keynote speaker, she's written numerous books and articles; her most recent book is a Berrett-Koehler bestseller, *Conversations Worth Having: Using Appreciative Inquiry to Fuel Productive and Meaningful Engagement*. She's been featured in leading media sources including *Fast Company, Forbes, HR Magazine, SmartBrief, Training Industry, and Training*

Magazine. Her keynote presentations reach a broad range of people, including HR Directors, organization development practitioners, women leaders, youth prevention specialists, educators, and individual social profit organizations and corporations. A perpetual learner, she's accumulated a Ph.D. in Collaborative Learning, an MBA, Masters in Transpersonal Psychology, Level II certification in the Barrett Values Cultural Assessment tools, and Level II certification in Spiral Dynamics Integral. cheri@conversationsworthhaving.today

Jackie Stavros, DM. Jackie's passion is working with others to discover their purpose in creating positive change. The heart of her work is using Appreciative Inquiry (AI), one of the most popular approaches to positive change that brings out the best in people to impact productivity, engagement, and performance. Jackie integrates strengths-based approaches into her research, training, coaching, and consulting work to strengthen relationships and inspire innovation. She has worked across all sectors, including for-profit, nonprofit, government, and a wide spectrum of industries. Jackie is a professor at Lawrence Technological University (LTU) College of Business and IT in Michigan. She is a member of the AI Council of Practitioners for the Cooperrider Center for Appreciative Inquiry and the Taos Institute. She serves as an Appreciative Inquiry Mentor for XCHANGE: Conversations for Exponential Growth. Before joining LTU, her industry work included manufacturing, automotive, banking, technology, government, and professional services.

Jackie has authored many books and articles, including: *Conversations Worth Having: Using Appreciative Inquiry to Fuel Productive and Meaningful Engagement, Appreciative Inquiry Handbook: For Leadership of Change* and *Learning to SOAR: Creating Strategy that Inspires Innovation and Engagement.* Her work has been featured in *Forbes, SmartBrief, Detroit's Live in the*

D, and *dbusiness Magazine.* She has presented her research and work in over 25 countries. Jackie earned a Doctorate in Management from Case Western Reserve University, an MBA from Michigan State University, and a BA from Wayne State University. jackie@conversationsworthhaving.today

Made in the USA
Columbia, SC
01 March 2023

13142663R20057